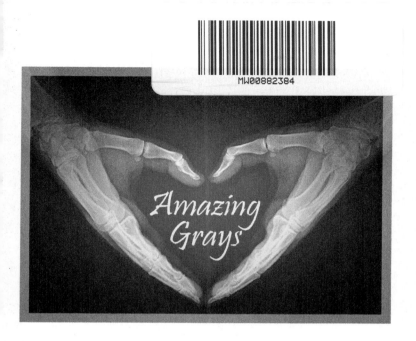

Amazing Grays

Spiritual reflections on the human body

By

Martha R. Hinman, PT, EdD

Illustrated by Maria del Carmen Cabrera

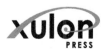

Table of Contents

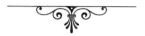

PREFACE

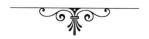

*I*n 1858, Dr. Henry Gray published the first edition of *Anatomy: Descriptive and Surgical* which was illustrated by fellow surgeon, Dr. Henry Vandyke Carter. Eighty years later, the book was officially retitled *Gray's Anatomy* and continued to be regarded as the most authoritative textbook on human anatomy. Generations of physicians and other health care professionals have "cut their teeth" in their academic training using this famous text which is still considered the most comprehensive and detailed book on the subject. Rare 1st editions of this classic now start at $3000 on eBay! The 40th edition of *Gray's Anatomy* was published in 2008, marking its 150th anniversary. In 2015, the 41st edition was released in a volume that contains 1,584 pages, weighs over 10 pounds, and is sold in both print and online versions. Few books have been published continuously for so many years without any decline in their popularity or application. Perhaps the longevity of this text may be attributed in part to the ageless nature of its subject matter. Despite ongoing scientific discoveries which continue to expand our understanding of how the human body works, the organism itself has remained essentially the same for thousands of years. That fact alone is rather amazing given the dramatic amount of change and evolution that has occurred in the world around us.

Although I make no attempt to mimic such a great literary feat as *Gray's Anatomy*, it is my hope that *Amazing Grays* will provide the reader with an opportunity to reflect on this same content from a spiritual, rather than a purely scientific, perspective. Although this book was originally intended for individuals who have dedicated their lives to the study and care of the human body, it should be of interest to anyone who is simply curious about the intricacies of our anatomical design or fascinated by little known details related to its function. Those of us who have studied the human body and marveled at its complexity cannot help being inspired by God's most wondrous creation. I hope these spiritual reflections will continue to feed that inspiration and serve as a reminder that we truly are *"fearfully and wonderfully made"*(Psalm 139:14)

Dr. Martha R. Hinman

DISCLAIMER

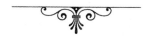

*T*he information in this book was derived from a variety of sources including encyclopedia, books, magazine and journal articles, and internet web sites. The author cannot validate the accuracy of all the information cited from these sources. Scriptural references were selected from the *New Century Version* of the Bible; thus, the wording may vary somewhat from that found in other Biblical sources.

DEDICATION

*N*o endeavor like this is ever completed without the support and encouragement of many people. I would like to first thank my parents, Richard and Lois Rammel, whose thirst for learning, commitment to service, and faith in God gave me the direction I needed to get this far in life. Though they are no longer living, their spiritual presence remains a strong source of my personal inspiration. As a physical therapist and teacher, I have also been inspired daily by the many patients, students, and colleagues I have been privileged to work with throughout my professional career. I am especially grateful to friends, Marsha Rutland, Jane Melton, and Nathan Tinkle who read this manuscript and offered editorial advice to ensure its accuracy and clarity. I am also fortunate to have met Carmen Cabrera, an angel with a palette, whose illustrations so vividly capture the inner beauty of the human body. Finally, I doubt this book would ever have been completed without the loving support and patience of my husband, Pete Hinman, Jr., who allowed me to borrow precious moments from our vacation time to put my thoughts in writing. His presence in my life has truly been my greatest joy and blessing.

1

Amazing Heredity

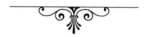

*D*eoxyribonucleic acid (DNA) is the sequence of genetic material, also known as a *genome*, which determines all of our physical traits. Every living cell with the exception of red blood cells contains strands of DNA that are arranged in the familiar, compact shape of a double helix. If all DNA in the human body were unwound it would reach to the moon and back 6,000 times! DNA was first discovered in 1869 by Friedrich Miescher, but it took another 144 years before scientists deciphered these DNA sequences as they worked on the Human Genome Project (HGP). This mapping project shed new light on the transmission of many hereditary conditions, some of which can have devastating effects on our quality of life or basic survival. It has also provided a means for manipulating gene sequences in order to eradicate these conditions and create "new and improved" versions of plants, animals, and humans. Of course, as with many scientific discoveries, this information has probably created more ethical controversies than practical solutions. First, there's the tremendous cost of the HGP which many critics believe is not a good use of limited research funding. Although the HGP has provided new diagnostic insights and capabilities, it has not produced any noteworthy treatments for those genetic conditions it has identified. Thus, a second source of criticism relates to the emotional distress this knowledge may create for individuals who are offered a diagnosis, but no cure. Conversely, supporters suggest that knowledge of defective genes may give couples the information needed to pursue other family planning options, and spare them the cost and stress of raising a child with a chronic illness or disability. Finally, many social, political, and religious groups have expressed concern over the manipulation of genetic material simply because science has made it possible. One has to wonder whether the results of such genetic engineering will ultimately produce unintended consequences that are far more harmful than beneficial. After all, if we were created by an all-knowing God, is it really a good idea to tinker with His blueprint?

I am the Lord. There is no other God; I am the only God. I will make you strong, even though you don't know me, so that everyone will know there is no other God. From the east to the west they will know I alone am the Lord. I made the light and the darkness. I bring peace, and I cause troubles. I, the Lord, do all these things (Isaiah 45:5-7).

2

Amazing Individuality

$\int$cientists tell us that all humans share more than 99% of the same genetic material, and we also share a significant amount with other species. For example, our DNA is 98% the same as a chimpanzee and 50% the same as the bananas that both species like to eat! And yet we know that each of us is also very unique. Apparently our distinct identity is determined by only 0.1% of our DNA. Although that may not sound like much, when we consider the fact that every inch of DNA contains about 25 GB of information, it seems to give God enough material to work with in making each human special. Another unique identifier is found in our fingerprints. These skin ridges on the tips of our fingers and thumbs provide friction and traction to manipulate objects, as well as enhance our sense of touch. Cats and dogs have similar types of prints on their noses. In humans, fingerprints develop during the 3rd month of fetal life and, unlike other physical features, they remain constant throughout our lifetime.

Hundreds of years ago, records from ancient China and Persia first documented the use of hand-prints as a means of personal identification. Today, finger-printing is used worldwide as the most common form of forensic evidence in criminal investigations. The three basic fingerprint patterns are the arch, the loop, and the whorl. Despite the commonality of these patterns, each human has a unique set of prints – even identical twins! Before the mid-1800s, law enforcement relied on officials who had extraordinary visual memories to identify previously arrested offenders by sight. Obviously this method led to many false arrests as individuals learned to alter their physical appearance. Around 1870, French anthropologist, Alphonse Bertillon, developed a more scientific identification system based on the dimensions of certain bony parts of the body which were applied to a formula. The Bertillon System was generally accepted for 30 years until the 1903 arrest of a man named Will West. As fate would have it, Will was sentenced to the penitentiary in Leavenworth, Kansas where another prisoner named William West was found to have identical Bertillon measurements. Thus, the two men were incorrectly identified as the same person until a fingerprint comparison revealed their distinct identities. Additional evidence later determined that the two men were actually twin brothers. Despite such similarities, there is little doubt that God intended for each of us to be a one-of-a-kind specimen. And although the Bible tells us that we are all created in His image, our individuality is reflected in our physical appearance, personality, talents, and life accomplishments – for God had something special in mind when he created human beings.

> *So God created human beings in his image. In the image of God he created them. He created them male and female. God blessed them and said, 'Have many children and grow in number. Fill the earth and be its master. Rule over the fish in the sea and over the birds in the sky and over every living thing that moves on the earth' (Genesis 1:27-28).*

3

Amazing Agility

*T*he encounter between David and Goliath is probably one of the best known and most cited stories of the Bible. The odds of David slaying such a formidable opponent with a stone delivered by a slingshot seems overwhelming and improbable to most of us. But many scholars believe that Goliath's size, estimated to be somewhere in the range of 9 to 10 feet tall, might actually have been attributed to a hormonal condition known as acromegaly. This condition is often caused by an adenoma (non-cancerous tumor) of the pituitary gland which causes an excessive secretion of growth hormone. Although once believed to be an acquired condition, recent evidence reported by Chahal and colleagues in a 2011 issue of the *New England Journal of Medicine* suggests that acromegaly may also be caused by a genetic mutation. Given other Biblical references to the large stature of some of Goliath's relatives, it is likely that his condition may have been inherited. In any case, we know that Goliath also had some visual impairment, probably due to the tumor's close proximity to, and pressure on, his optic nerve. In addition, someone of Goliath's size is not likely to move as quickly, nor be as agile, as someone who is David's size. Nerve impulses travel at a certain velocity (40-50 meters/second) regardless of one's height. Goliath's nerves would have further to travel given his longer limbs; thus, his movement time was likely to be much slower than David's. So perhaps David had a more strategic advantage than he realized when he engaged the giant in this deadly duel. Likewise, we often tend to overlook the advantages God has given us to take on the "giants" in our lives. So whether we are facing the challenge of a difficult exam or caring for someone with a terminal diagnosis, we can overcome any adversity if we're willing to trust Him enough to pick up that slingshot!

You gave me strength in battle. You made my enemies bow before me" (Psalm 18:39).

4

Amazing Velocity

*O*n April 26, 2009, French swimmer Frédérick Bousquet set a new world record in the 50-meter freestyle with a time of 20.94 seconds, making his average swim speed a little over 5 mph. So how does this compare to the swimming speed of the millions of sperm which are racing to reach that prized egg while it is still viable? The answer is about 5 mm per second. Given their minute size of only .002 inches from head to tail, this means sperm can travel about 0.2 inch per second. Although this might not sound too fast, when compared to the size of other species, a sperm's speed would be equivalent to a salmon swimming about 500 miles an hour or a whale doing 15,000 miles an hour in open water. So these sexy little swimmers are certainly swift! But given the brief window of time for fertilization to occur, they must also have a good sense of direction. So how do these blind and brainless sperm find their way to a single egg that is still hidden inside a tiny fallopian tube? According to a 2003 study published by the Weizmann Institute, sperm are like tiny heat-seeking missiles that initially follow a thermal gradient from their entry point in the vagina to the warmer temperature found in the fallopian tubes. The term for this process is *thermotaxis*. After they find the fallopian tube containing the egg and gain entry into its warmer environment, the remaining sperm can pick up the egg's scent like a miniature pack of hound dogs. This attraction is caused by the release of chemicals from the egg itself which attract these eager sperm through a process known as *chemotaxis*. Upon reaching their intended target, the surviving sperm release a flurry of enzymes that peck away at the egg's layered shell until one lucky swimmer penetrates the final protective coating and completes the fertilization process. Millions of other sperm die along the way, but for one that makes it, the reward is great! Given these incredible odds, it seems clear that divine intervention is needed to complete each act of fertilization. Similar to the direction God gives these tiny sperm, Christ assures the success of our endeavors if we are first willing to seek His guidance.

Ask, and God will give to you. Search, and you will find. Knock, and the door will open for you" (Matthew 7:7).

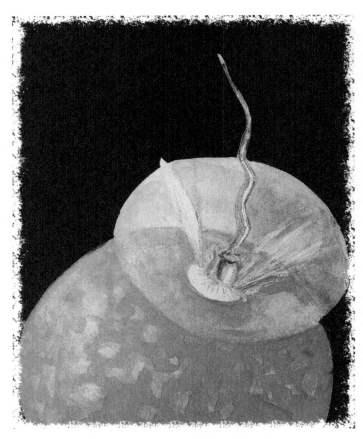

The body's architects

5

Amazing Creativity

$\mathcal{U}$nlike her male counterpart who creates millions of new sperm on a daily basis, the female human is born with all her eggs in one basket – or should we say two baskets, given her pair of ovaries. Before she is ever born, the female body has already created millions of egg cells, or *ova*, to ensure her ability to reproduce later in life. These little baskets of miracles still number 2 million ova at the time of birth, but by puberty that number has diminished to about 400,000. Each month thousands of immature ova die, leaving only a few to mature and eventually be released during ovulation. These eggs, the size of a pinhead, are actually the largest single cell in the human body and the only one that is visible to the naked eye. And they have great expectations to go along with their size! If a lucky sperm finds and penetrates that egg's shell during the 24 hours after its release, their union produces the world's next human. The miracle of conception also creates great expectations for most parents, who wonder what this child will look like, how it will behave, and what it will accomplish as he or she grows. Likewise, our heavenly Father expectantly watches us develop from this tiny egg into a mature human and probably marvels at the uniqueness of each of His creations, no two of which are exactly alike, not even identical twins. And although He chose to give each of us each a special identity and purpose in this life, the Book of Psalms tells us that He knows what course our lives will take even before we draw our first breath. How blessed we are to have a Creator who so carefully planned the purpose and function of our every cell!

You made my whole being; you formed me in my mother's body. I praise you because you made me in an amazing and wonderful way. What you have done is wonderful. I know this very well. You saw my bones being formed as I took shape in my mother's body. When I was put together there, you saw my body as it was formed. All the days planned for me were written in your book before I was one day old (Psalm 139:13-16).

6

Amazing Sexuality

If men and women were both asked to describe the primary purpose of the breast, they would likely give very different answers. However, if we combined their responses, we would probably come up with three important functions: (1) they nourish an infant; (2) they help shape a woman's body image, and (3) they are a source of erotic pleasure. Of the many references to the breast that are made in the Bible, those in the Song of Solomon are definitely the most descriptive. Here, the breasts of Solomon's lover are vividly described as "two fawns," "twin gazelles," "clusters of grapes," and "towers." We certainly get the impression that this woman was well endowed! Despite variations in the size and shape of women's breasts (a trait that is unique to the human species), the woman who sets the Guinness record for having the largest natural breasts is Annie Hawkins-Turner whose chest circumference is approximately 70 inches. These measurements would put her in a size 48-V bra, which is not currently manufactured, so she must squeeze into a smaller size 52-I. Born in 1958, Annie is 5 feet and 6 inches tall and weighs about 350 pounds; approximately 1/3 of this body weight is carried in her breast tissue.

So big or small, what type of tissue are we talking about here? According to an article published by the Sinclair Intimacy Institute, the female breast is comprised of 15 to 25 milk-producing glands, which are connected to milk ducts that converge inside the nipple. The remainder of the breast is fat and fibrous connective tissue that binds the breast together and gives it shape. Nipples, which come in their own variety of shapes and colors, are blessed with an abundance of nerve endings, making them particularly sensitive to touch. They also contain thin muscle fibers which enable them to become stiff and erect when stimulated. A 2011 study published in *The Journal of Sexual Medicine* provided evidence of a direct neurological connection between nipple stimulation and perceived genital arousal. These findings were based on multiple functional MRI scans in which the genital areas of each woman's cerebral cortex were activated whenever her nipples were stimulated. These findings came as a surprise to the male investigators but not to most women who have known about this erotic connection for years! Nevertheless, it was nice to finally have some scientific validation. Obviously God designed some hidden circuitry in a woman's nervous system that He intended for her mate to discover and enjoy.

You are beautiful and pleasant; my love, you are full of delights. You are tall like a palm tree, and your breasts are like its bunches of fruit. I said, 'I will climb up the palm tree and take hold of its fruit' (Song of Solomon 7:6-8).

7

Amazing Versatility

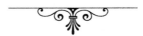

*H*ave you ever wondered why babies put so many objects in their mouth? Or why we experience such intense pain when we accidentally bite our tongue? Or why a "French kiss" can be so stimulating? Besides its unique function as a sensory organ for taste, the nerve endings on the tongue are also extremely sensitive to touch. In fact, it is the first sense to develop in utero. Babies develop their sense of touch in the lips and mouth at only 8 weeks gestation. In addition to being a sensory organ, the tongue is the only muscle in the body that is not attached at both ends. This anatomic distinction gives the tongue the unique ability to use its motor function to further explore the size, shape, and texture of objects it comes in contact with. The tongue's maneuverability is also what allows us to formulate the words needed to articulate our thoughts, feelings, and ideas. Thus, the tongue is capable of sensing, moving, and communicating like no other structure in the body. Despite its agility and sensitivity, the tongue's liability is when it speaks without civility! In fact the Bible makes about 150 references to the tongue, particularly in the Books of Psalms and Proverbs, where we are admonished to speak with caution, because our words can reflect our true nature and intentions.

In addition to its versatile talents, the tongue's appearance can also serve as a gauge of our overall health through changes in its color, size, and texture. For example, a healthy tongue is usually pink, whereas a purple or bluish tongue may be associated with poor circulation. Red or yellow tongues may indicate a bacterial infection while white patches could signify a fungus. Swollen tongues are typically associated with an acute allergic reaction, and a furry tongue may indicate a gastrointestinal problem such as constipation. And what does a black hairy-looking tongue mean? Either a big spider has just crawled into that person's mouth, or they may have a yeast infection, diabetes, or simply poor oral hygiene. So, if you are a health care provider, it pays to listen to your patient's tongue – in more ways than one!

Lord, help me control my tongue; help me be careful about what I say. Take away my desire to do evil or to join others in doing wrong. Don't let me eat tasty food with those who do evil (Psalm 141:3-4).

8

Amazing Adaptability

*B*abies are born with 300 bones, but by adulthood we have only 206 in our bodies. So what happens to the other 94 bones? They don't really disappear, they just fuse together. For example, the bones of the cranium and the pelvis are moveable in a baby to facilitate the delivery process, but they eventually form a tight, stable connection via fibrous tissue and function as a single bone. Anatomists still label most of these as separate bones, so it really depends on how we want to count them. For example, the 8 bones of the cranium that enclose and protect the brain include the sphenoid, occipital, frontal, parietal, temporal, and ethmoid bones. The occipital bone is in the back and the frontal bone, naturally, is in the front. The two sides of the cranium consist of the upper parietal bones and the lower temporal bones, while the sphenoid connects these other six bones from the inside. Between the eye sockets lies the ethmoid bone which separates the nasal cavity from the brain. Fourteen additional bones form the underlying structure of the face and only one of these, the mandible (lower jaw), is moveable. In adults, all the rest of these bones are fused together by interlocking joints called *sutures*. So we don't really lose any skeletal parts as we grow; they just tend to become more rigid.

Unfortunately, many of us allow the same thing to happen to our minds. Maybe that's why the term "bonehead" is such a good descriptor for our sometimes narrow-minded behavior! However, even though our skulls have a rigid exterior, the brain it houses has an extremely adaptable quality known as *plasticity*. This characteristic is what allows us to continuously reorganize our brain's structure and function as we learn new behaviors, store a lifetime of memories, and attempt to compensate for damaged neural pathways. This capacity to grow and evolve as a human being is a powerful gift. Hopefully, we will use it as wisely as King Solomon did!

God gave Solomon great wisdom so he could understand many things. His wisdom was as hard to measure as the grains of sand on the seashore. His wisdom was greater than any wisdom of the East, or any wisdom in Egypt (1 Kings 4:29-30).

9

Amazing Density

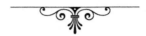

In 1895, German physicist, Wilhelm Röentgen's accidental discovery of x-ray radiation revolutionized medicine by giving physicians the ability to peer inside the human body to diagnose a variety of skeletal and soft tissue abnormalities, as well as locate foreign objects such as metal shrapnel. These insightful rays often expose the source of symptoms that were previously unexplained. As an example, the cover photo of this book revealed a small bone fragment at the base of the author's left thumb that has caused intermittent pain which she previously attributed to an arthritic joint. Take another look – can you see it? X-rays are designed to reflect the density of the tissues that the radiation penetrates. The greater the tissue's density, the more radiation it absorbs, creating a relatively opaque (white) appearance. However, less dense structures and those filled with air (like healthy lungs)

allow more radiation to pass through; thus they appear as darker shades of gray or black on an x-ray. When we are born, our bones are not fully calcified, but rather are primarily composed of cartilage. This gives the infant the flexibility it needs to navigate through the birth canal. As the child grows, his or her skeleton gradually becomes more calcified until it fully matures in the third decade of life. But bone is a living, growing tissue that is constantly changing. Normal "wear and tear" causes bone to break down and rebuild itself through a process known as *remodeling*. This process isn't much different than that which occurs when we remodel our home. The foundation remains intact as does most of the home's outer shell, but outdated interior structures are removed and replaced with newer ones. Bone remodeling occurs at a more rapid pace in young children and progressively slows as we age. Thus, a child's skeleton may turnover as often as every 6 months, while an adult's skeleton requires a couple years to completely remodel. Several factors facilitate bone remodeling including hormonal stimulation, adequate nutrition, and physical stresses applied via muscle contractions and weight-bearing. The stimulation of bone-growing cells called *osteoblasts*, by physical stress is known as Wolff's Law. Thus, the more active we are throughout our lifetime, the stronger our bones will be when we get older. This is important because we begin to lose bone density and strength as early as age 35. As these bones become more porous, their x-ray appearance changes from bright white to shades of gray. In cases of severe bone loss, (a.k.a., *osteoporosis*) portions of the bone may no longer be visible on x-ray at all. Although osteoporosis typically occurs later in life, some people develop this bone disease in response to other pathology or treatment such as chemotherapy and corticosteroid drugs. The spinal vertebrae, neck of the femur (hip), and distal end of the radius (wrist) are particularly prone to osteoporosis and become common sites for fragility fractures as we age. To avoid this fate, we must discourage bad habits in our youth such as sedentary behavior, cigarette smoking, and a diet that lacks sufficient bone nutrients like calcium and vitamin D. Remember, we reap what we sow, and our bones know that quite well. So put this book down for a while, take a brisk walk, and refresh yourself with a glass of cold milk!

My life is ending in sadness, and my years are spent in crying. My troubles are using up my strength, and my bones are getting weaker (Psalm 31:10).

10

Amazing Vulnerability

*T*he femur is known as the biggest and strongest bone in the human body. Its ball-shaped head articulates with the socket of the hip (the acetabulum), and its rounded condyles at the bottom help form the hinge of the knee joint. Thus, the femur provides a long lever for transmitting the weight of our upper body down to the base of support at our feet. Its massive size allows it to resist forces of 2000 pounds or more. Yet, like many objects of great size and strength, it does have a weak link. The angle formed between the head and shaft of the femur is referred to as the femoral neck, and within the neck is a region known as *Ward's triangle*. Due to the architecture of its bony matrix, this section of the femur normally has only 70% of the strength found in the rest of the bone, and that proportion diminishes with age. When someone twists and falls, the torque is typically transmitted through this area of the bone, often resulting in a femoral neck fracture. More commonly, we refer to this injury as a hip fracture. Years ago, people who sustained this type of fracture were placed in bed traction for several months, a treatment that was fraught with risks associated with prolonged immobilization. Death from complications such as bone infections and pneumonia was not uncommon. However, since the development of prosthetic joint implants in the 1960s, surgical treatment has become the standard care for hip fractures. The procedure for replacing the broken end of the femur (and often the socket it articulates with) is known as *hip arthroplasty*, and it has dramatically reduced both the morbidity and mortality associated with hip fractures. Although surgery is not without risks, especially for elderly patients, this procedure allows earlier mobilization and weight-bearing for the patient and is more likely to restore functional mobility. Despite these medical advancements, we still have not made much progress in reducing the incidence of these life-threatening fractures. Approximately 1/3 of older adults in the U.S. fall each year and recent statistics indicate that more than ¼ million of them will require treatment for hip fractures at a cost ranging from $10.3 to $15.2 billion. By 2050, the annual number of hip fractures in the U.S. is expected to at least double – perhaps even quadruple – while worldwide estimates are projected to exceed 6 million![1] Isn't it amazing how such a small slice of bone can have such a staggering impact? Perhaps Ward's triangle should remind

---

[1] http://www.uptodate.com/contents/total-hip-arthroplasty

us that we are only as strong as our weakest link. Thus, none of us can provide these patients, or any others, with the best care if we try to act alone. But when we work together, we can compensate for each other's limitations and provide a quality of care that ensures a better outcome.

Two people are better than one, because they get more done by working together. If one falls down, the other can help him up. But it is bad for the person who is alone and falls, because no one is there to help (Ecclesiastes 4:9-10).

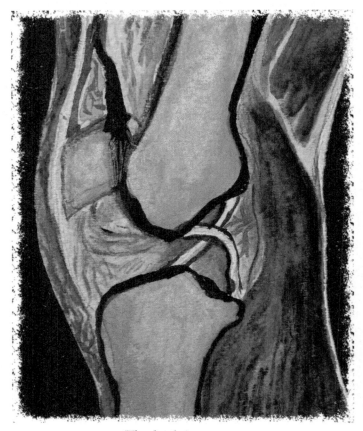

The body's movers

11

Amazing Synchrony

You ou may have heard someone who has jaw trouble
say, "I have TMJ," which is technically incor-
rect for two reasons. First, the term TMJ refers to the
temporomandibular joint which is an anatomical structure, not a disorder. Secondly, God gave us two TMJs,
not just one. What is unique about this pair of joints is
that they are connected by a single bone which makes
their movements virtually inseparable. As far as joints
are concerned, these two function like Siamese twins!
Furthermore, they probably move more often than any
other joint in the body – every time we talk, chew, or
yawn. So if we are a hungry, sleepy, jabber box, our
TMJs will get quite a workout! Normally when we
open our mouth, the mandible drops down as its upper
ends roll and glide forward in their sockets. If you
were to place your fingers in your ears (or right in front
of them) you would feel these joints move when you

open and close your own mouth. Because the TMJs are fairly loose joints and undergo such frequent movement, they are highly susceptible to dysfunction which is commonly referred to as *temporomandibular disorder,* or *TMD.* There are many things that can affect the synchronous function of the TMJs including poor posture, abnormal alignment of the teeth, facial trauma, arthritis, and even excessive chewing. The National Institute of Dental and Craniofacial Research estimates that as many as 10 million Americans probably suffer from some type of TMD.

Nevertheless, the collaborative motion of these joints should remind us of the importance of working together as a health care team. If one of us becomes dysfunctional, it is likely to affect the rest of the team and make our overall patient care plan ineffective, perhaps even harmful, for the patient. The importance of interprofessional collaboration (IPC) is eloquently stated by Dr. Peter Pronovost in his book entitled *Safe Patients, Smart Hospitals* where he acknowledges the following:

"Yet few medical and nursing programs train students in how to work effectively in teams, despite a wealth of evidence that has shown this is key to improving safety and quality of care. When I was in medical school I spent hundreds of hours looking into a microscope – a skill I never needed to know or ever use. Yet I didn't have a single class that taught me

communication and teamwork skills – some-thing I need every day I walk into the hos-pital." (p. 46)

Fortunately, TMD is treated fairly easily, and the collaborative effort of health care teams is also attainable. The first condition usually responds well to exercise and oral orthotics. The prescription for the latter condition includes a simple resection of the ego followed by an injection of humility, and a maintenance dose of respect.

Always be humble, gentle, and patient, accepting each other in love. You are joined together with peace through the Spirit, so make every effort to continue together in this way. There is one body and one Spirit, and God called you to have one hope. There is one Lord, one faith, and one baptism. There is one God and Father of everything. He rules every-thing and is everywhere and is in everything (Ephesians 4:2-6).

12

Amazing Flexibility

*D*o you recall the story of Joshua and the Battle of Jericho? The city was protected by a strong wall that appeared to be impenetrable. But God devised a plan for Joshua to bring down the wall and destroy the city through several days of marching around it while shouting and blowing trumpets. Could the acoustic vibrations alone have been sufficient to bring down such a solid wall without God's divine intervention? Surely not. Yet this story reminds us that even the most secure structures can be vulnerable to minor stresses if they develop a weakness. The spinal column is one of those structures. It is actually a rather precarious stack of 24 blocks of bone called vertebrae that sit atop a narrow wedge called the sacrum. They are separated by shock-absorbing cushions known as intervertebral disks and bound together by a series of ligaments and muscles of varying lengths. With the exception of the first two vertebrae in the neck, only a small amount of gliding motion occurs between each vertebral segment. Yet when their efforts are combined, the spine can bend, straighten, or twist in just about any direction. Sounds like a well-designed team, doesn't it? Of course, like any team, when one member fails to do his job, the work of the entire team may be in jeopardy. In the case of the spine, the most common culprit is an intervertebral disk, usually one in the lower back. These disks are comprised of a central portion, the nucleus pulposus (NP), which is very fluid, much like jelly or toothpaste, and moves when we bend in various directions. If we placed a rubber ball between two boards and squeezed them together, we could easily simulate the movement of these disks. The outer cartilaginous ring *(annulus fibrosis)* normally contains the NP when it is placed under pressure. But these annular rings can fray over time, just like an old rope or electrical wire, creating a weakness in the disk's fibrous wall. Although a healthy disk can withstand repetitive forces of high magnitudes such as those produced by a power weight lifter, a degenerative disk can rupture under minimal loading just as the wall of Jericho crumbled to the mere sound of a trumpet. When the NP pushes beyond the bounds of the weakened annulus, it produces a herniated or "slipped" disk. Once it escapes, that wayward disk typically runs into one of the spinal nerves that emerge between each pair of vertebrae. Ouch – those nerves do not like pressure! They also carry nerve impulses to and from our extremities, so prolonged pressure from a protruding disk can cause numbness and weakness in an arm or leg. If you are one of the 75% of people who has experienced back pain, you know how debilitating this condition can be. Fortunately many disk problems can be treated non-surgically using a variety of traction and manipulation techniques that have been practiced in some form for nearly 5000 years. According to Dr. Freddy Kaltenborn, a leading expert in spinal manipulative therapy, one of the earliest traction treatments for the spine was the "falling ladder" maneuver. A patient was fastened to a ladder that was raised and then suddenly dropped, producing a general thrust force through the entire spine. Fortunately, our contemporary traction and manipulation techniques are much safer and more refined than the falling ladder! These manual therapy techniques are now integrated into the education and practice of many health care professionals including physical therapists, osteopathic physicians, and chiropractors. But the best treatment is always prevention. Learning to maintain good posture, use proper lifting techniques, and engage in regular exercise will keep our spine strong and able to withstand life's minor stresses, including the sound of a trumpet!

When the priests blew the trumpets, the people shouted. At the sound of the trumpets and the people's shout, the walls fell, and everyone ran straight into the city. So the Israelites defeated that city (Joshua 6:20).

13

Amazing Utility

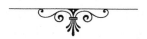

*H*ere's a riddle: *"We aren't visible in newborns and may disappear when you're old, but in between you will see us whenever lips unfold."* Yes, of course – the answer is our teeth! As everyone knows, we are born with two sets of teeth. The first 20 "baby teeth" begin erupting in pairs around 6 months of age, starting with the centrally-located incisors. After age 4, the bones of the face and jaw begin to grow which creates more space between this first set of teeth. Around age 6 or 7, we start shedding our temporary teeth and replacing them with a set of 32 permanent, adult teeth. From front to back we should end up with a pair of central incisors, a pair of lateral incisors, a pair of cuspids (or canines), two pairs of bicuspids (or premolars), and 3 pairs of molars. The 3rd set of molars, also known as the "wisdom teeth," are somewhat variable in terms of their eruption and are often removed due to poor alignment or impaction. Obviously, the shape of these different types of teeth makes each of them suited for a different purpose. The incisors are good for biting, the cuspids and bicuspids help tear food apart, and the molars grind it into smaller pieces that can be easily swallowed and digested.

Not only do these chompers come in handy when it's time to eat, but they are also one of our most noticeable physical features. Recent surveys indicate that 50% of people claim the first physical feature they notice in another person is his or her smile. And that smile makes the most lasting impression! In addition, most people are willing to invest in procedures to maintain the quality of their teeth. According to the Centers for Medicare and Medicaid, Americans spent $111 billion on dental care in 2013; nearly $3 million of that amount was spent on cosmetic procedures such as teeth straightening or whitening. Although the enameled surface of our teeth is the toughest material in the human body, like all other body parts, it can eventually wear out. Rather than resorting to the consumption of soft food, civilizations over the years have found creative ways to replace lost teeth. As early as 700 BC, the Etruscans of Northern Italy fashioned primitive dentures from the discarded teeth of humans and animals. Beginning in the 18th century AD, dentures were fabricated from materials such as animal ivory, porcelain, and gold, along with teeth extracted from fallen soldiers on the battlefield. Despite popular belief, George Washington's false teeth were not made of wood, but rather a plate of carved hippopotamus ivory that was inlaid with teeth from horses, donkeys, and humans. Of course, modern materials such as acrylic resin and plastic are now used to produce customized replicas that are far more durable and attractive than any of their predecessors. So regardless of how old we get or how many teeth we lose, we can still retain our most endearing physical feature – our smile!

Your teeth are white like newly sheared sheep just coming from their bath. Each one has a twin, and none of them is missing (Song of Solomon 4:2).

14

Amazing Regularity

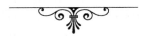

*O*ur bodies contain three types of muscle tissue. *Skeletal muscles*, which have a striated appearance, are the most familiar to us because we have voluntary control over when and how hard they work to produce movement. The heart is composed of its own distinct type of muscle known as *cardiac muscle*; its sole purpose is to serve as a pump for our circulatory system. Although only a few people can learn to consciously control the rate at which their heart muscle contracts, all of us are aware of its beating sensation. The third type is *smooth muscle* which lines our blood vessels, airway, digestive tract, and bladder. These muscles work very subtly, without conscious awareness or control, giving new meaning to the term "smooth operators." Like a well-rehearsed orchestra, they time their contractions to sequentially move food from one end to the other through a process known as *peristalsis.* These muscles are strong enough to move food through the gut regardless of what position our body is in or other activity we are engaged in. Although food usually travels on a one-way highway through our esophagus, stomach, and intestinal tract, when we get extremely nauseated this process can reverse itself. Most of us are familiar with this unpleasant act known as *emesis.* Of course, people use a variety of more common terms to describe this physiological phenomenon such as vomiting, puking, heaving, hurling, upchucking, barfing, and tossing your cookies. Regardless of what we call it, this forceful ejection of partially digested food is actually a coordinated effort involving several muscle groups. First, the deep muscles of inspiration create a negative thoracic pressure, while the abdominal muscles create a positive abdominal pressure. Next, the smooth muscles in the esophagus and stomach undergo reverse peristalsis, while the esophageal sphincter undergoes relaxation. The unpleasant odor associated with vomit is attributed to high levels of butyric acid, which interestingly, is also a concentrated ingredient in parmesan cheese. When blindfolded, most people cannot even tell the difference between the two! But an astute nose can smell the difference, just as God can detect someone whose faith and actions are insincere. So let's keep the "smooth operators" inside our bodies, and strive to be wholly genuine on the outside.

Create in me a pure heart, God, and make my spirit right again (Psalm 51:10).

15

Amazing Reliability

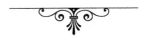

*M*easuring about one millimeter in size, the *stapedius* muscle distinguishes itself as the smallest in the human body. This tiny muscle is located in the tympanic cavity of the middle ear and attaches to the neck of the smallest bone, the *stapes*. Because of its horseshoe-shaped appearance, the stapes is sometimes called the stirrup. When a loud sound is heard, the stapedius muscle reflexively pulls on the head of the stapes to reduce excess vibration and protect the inner ear from damage. If a loud or lengthy sound is heard, such as a gun firing or a rock band playing, the stapedius pulls the stapes away from the cochlea, the portion of the ear that enables us to hear. Likewise, the tensor tympani muscle pulls on the malleus (a.k.a. "the hammer") which facilitates the transmission of sound waves. This phenomenon is known as the *acoustic reflex*. In addition, the muscle is responsible for another reflex, the *stapedius reflex*, which occurs when people speak. This reflex reduces inner-ear vibration and decreases the sound level heard by 20 decibels. If the stapedius did not perform so reliably, would could not tolerate the sound of our own voices. So the stapedius not only protects us from harmful sounds in our external environment – it also protects us from our own inner noise! As we are told in the Book of Proverbs, small things are not always strong and powerful, but their resourcefulness ensures their survival. The cleverly designed stapedius muscle could certainly be added to this list.

There are four things on earth that are small, but they are very wise: Ants are not very strong, but they store up food in the summer. Rock badgers are not very powerful, but they can live among the rocks. Locusts have no king, but they all go forward in formation. Lizards can be caught in the hand, but they are found even in kings' palaces (Proverbs 30:24-28).

16

Amazing Mobility

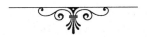

*S*o if the stapedius is the smallest muscle, which one gets the prize for being largest? If you guessed the one you're sitting on, you would be right! The *gluteus maximus*, or buttock muscle, makes up about 16% of the total cross-sectional muscle mass around the hip joint. Along with its cousins, the gluteus medius and minimus, this muscle controls most of the hip motions needed for us to stand up and walk. In addition, the gluteus maximus can claim more nicknames than any other muscle in the body. Among the many terms used to describe this portion of our anatomy are buttocks, bottom, derrière, cheeks, rear end, backside, keister, tush, buns, caboose, rump, fanny, heinie, ass, bum, butt, and the most recent label – booty. It seems the gluteus maximus has become the most popular muscle in American culture as women selectively enhance its size through vigorous exercise, silicone implants, and fat injections in hopes of developing a "sexy booty" that will attract the opposite sex. A quick online search revealed more than 50 books devoted solely to the development of larger buttocks! Although we may not understand the sudden fascination with gluteal enhancement, it is probably safe to assume that this fad, like most others, will fade over time. Because, as the writer of Ecclesiastes reminds us, there's a time for everything. And you can bet your bottom dollar on that!

There is a time for everything, and everything on earth has its special season. There is a time to be born and a time to die. There is a time to plant and a time to pull up plants. There is a time to kill and a time to heal. There is a time to destroy and a time to build. There is a time to cry and a time to laugh. There is a time to be sad and a time to dance. There is a time to throw away stones and a time to gather them. There is a time to hug and a time not to hug. There is a time to look for something and a time to stop looking for it. There is a time to keep things and a time to throw things away. There is a time to tear apart and a time to sew together. There is a time to be silent and a time to speak. There is a time to love and a time to hate. There is a time for war and a time for peace (Ecclesiastes 3:1-8).

17

Amazing Elasticity

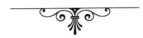

*T*endons and ligaments are commonly referred to as connective tissue because that's their job – to form connections between other structures. Tendons join muscle to bone, while ligaments secure the bony articulations at each joint. When dissecting a cadaver, the glistening white appearance of these connective tissues makes them some of the most beautiful structures in the human body. They are also uniquely equipped to provide both strength and flexibility to the connections they form. This characteristic is technically referred to as their *viscoelastic property*. Whenever we watch a skilled gymnast, dancer, or acrobat perform, we can appreciate the strength and flexibility of these tissues. And yet, they do have their limits! Weightlifters have sustained complete ruptures of their biceps and quadriceps tendons while attempting to set world records. Likewise, many athletes have been sidelined by ligamentous tears in their ankles, knees, and shoulders. This breaking point is referred to as the tendon or ligament's *tensile strength* – the point at which the tissue can no longer stretch or withstand any additional load without breaking. The tensile strength of tendons and ligaments varies according to their size and the individual's age – the older we get, the more brittle these structures become.

The thickest and longest tendon in the human body is the Achilles tendon which connects the calf muscles to the calcaneus (heel bone) of the foot. This tendon gets its name from the ancient Greek warrior, Achilles. You may recall that when Achilles was a baby, his mother dipped him in the river Styx which separated the lands of the dead and the living. This immersion gave Achilles great power, strength, and immortality. However, his mother held him by the heel when she performed this protective act which, of course, left that one body part unprotected. Alas, Achilles loses his life in battle during the Trojan War when an enemy's poison arrow strikes him through the tendon of that heel. Achilles' *one* weakness is still cited today as a pneumonic for remembering that the reflex activity associated with tapping the heel cord is controlled by the first sacral (*S1*) nerve root of the spine. More importantly, Achilles' story teaches us about the vulnerability of the human body, despite the use of training programs and protective equipment. Like our tendons and ligaments, we all have limitations, even though we may not always be aware of what those limitations are. Fortunately, we have surgeons who can repair torn tendons and ligaments when we exceed their tensile strength. And when we reach the limits of our spiritual strength, we have the Holy Spirit to intervene on our behalf.

Also, the Spirit helps us with our weakness. We do not know how to pray as we should. But the Spirit himself speaks to God for us, even begs God for us with deep feelings that words cannot explain. God can see what is in people's hearts. And he knows what is in the mind of the Spirit, because the Spirit speaks to God for his people in the way God wants. We know that in everything God works for the good of those who love him. They are the people he called, because that was his plan (Romans 8:26-28).

18

Amazing Dependability

*M*ankind has developed several pretty reliable delivery services such as UPS and FedEx, but none of them come close to matching the efficiency and dependability of the cardiovascular system which delivers life-sustaining oxygen and other nutrients to every other organ and tissue in the human body. Each drop of blood contains millions of tiny red blood cells (RBCs) which are produced by the bone marrow. These RBCs only live about 4 months, but during their short lifetime they make about 250,000 trips around our body (~ 12,000 miles a day) before they die. Powered by the left side of the heart, these little speed demons can circulate through the entire body in about one minute. When the oxygen-depleted blood returns to the heart, its right side pumps this blood back to the lungs to pick up more oxygen, a shorter journey requiring less than 10 seconds. If that speed isn't impressive enough, consider the incredible size of this vascular network. If we could extract all the blood vessels from the body and lay them end-to-end, they would measure more than 60,000 miles in length! That's equivalent to about 2½ trips around the globe. And unlike any other delivery service, this one operates 24/7 with no breaks or holidays. It literally never misses a beat! Don't you wish other delivery services were as dependable as the one God gave us? We should be grateful that the love He delivers lasts a lot longer than the life of a RBC!

So know that the Lord your God is God, the faithful God. He will keep his agreement of love for a thousand lifetimes for people who love him and obey his commands (Deuteronomy 7:9).

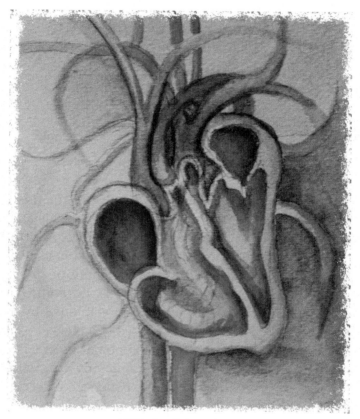

The body's pump

19

Amazing Fragility

*E*veryone knows that heart attacks can be fatal, but can someone actually die of a broken heart? The answer is "yes," although the actual odds of such an event are fairly low. Broken heart syndrome, also known as stress-induced cardiomyopathy or *takotsubo cardiomyopathy* (TCM or TTM), differs from a heart attack in that it is usually precipitated by a surge of stress hormones as opposed to a blockage in one or more coronary arteries. Although its precise cause is unknown, TCM most commonly occurs in women over age 50 who have experienced extreme physical or emotional trauma; it can also occur as a reaction to certain types of drugs. Because the symptoms of chest pain and shortness of breath mimic those of myocardial infarction, TCM is frequently misdiagnosed. However, unlike coronary artery disease, TCM is easily treated and most patients make a complete recovery without any lasting complications. And yet a 2014 meta-analysis published by Singh and colleagues in *The American Journal of Cardiology* reported a 4.5% mortality rate among patients who were hospitalized for TCM, suggesting that this condition is not as benign as some previously believed it to be.

So where does the name *"takotsubo"* come from? When the condition was first described by Japanese physicians in 1991, they noted the ballooning in the heart's apex (lower tip) on imaging tests which they thought resembled an ancient Japanese octopus trap called tako-tsubo. Who knew that an octopus trap and a broken heart had so much in common? However, it isn't hard to imagine that when an ocuptus gets caught in a tako-tsubo, it probably feels just as stressed as the individual who experiences an episode of TCM! Fortunately, the prognosis for an individual with TCM is far more optimistic than it is for the octopus, because we are blessed with a Great Physician who can comfort and heal us when we truly experience a broken heart, either physically or emotionally.

> ...*God lives forever and is holy. He is high and lifted up. He says, 'I live in a high and holy place, but I also live with people who are sad and humble. I give new life to those who are humble and to those whose hearts are broken'* (*Isaiah 57:15*).

20

Amazing Productivity

*A*lthough God gave us a single version of most internal organs, He must have had a good reason for giving us two kidneys. Perhaps He knew that the high volume of work required by these small, bean-shaped organs would cause them to wear out before many other body parts. Each day the kidneys filter the body's entire volume of blood (approximately 5½ liters) about 400 times through 140 miles of tubes and millions of tiny filters known as *nephrons*. Each nephron is comprised of a tuft of small blood vessels called the glomerulus which act as tiny sieves to remove the impurities from our blood and carry them away via the attached renal tubule. Given the compact size of the kidney (about 4½ inches long), there's a lot of cleaning that goes on inside such a small space! And despite the fact that the kidneys account for only 0.5% of the entire body weight, their arterial blood supply is greater than that received by the heart, brain, or liver; together they receive approximately 25% of the total blood volume pumped by the heart. Although a healthy person can live just as long with a single kidney, it's always nice to have a back-up organ, given that 1 in 3 Americans are at risk for developing kidney disease, the 9th leading cause of death in the U.S. According to the National Kidney Foundation, most of the 26 million Americans who have kidney disease don't even realize it. Common risk factors include high blood pressure, diabetes, family history, smoking, and cardiovascular disease. And, of course, there's the effect of aging. We tend to lose about 1% of our nephrons each year beginning around age 40. As a result, kidney failure is not an uncommon condition among the elderly. To avoid death from a gradual poisoning of our blood, artificial means of filtration known as *dialysis* may be used to substitute for failing kidneys until a suitable donor organ can be found. Despite the high frequency and success rate of kidney transplantation, the latest government data indicate that more than 101,000 of the 123,000 Americans who are currently on the organ transplant wait list need a kidney. Yet, fewer than 17,000 a year will receive one which means that before you finish reading this page, another person on that wait list has probably died. Nevertheless, it is reassuring to know that when our body fails in its ability to rid us of our physical impurities, we can still be cleansed spiritually through power of God's grace.

How much more is done by the blood of Christ. He offered himself through the eternal Spirit as a perfect sacrifice to God. His blood will make our consciences pure from useless acts so we may serve the living God (Hebrews 9:14).

21

Amazing Rigidity

*M*ost people are familiar with the term "hardening of the arteries" and "stiffening of the joints," two degenerative conditions that are often associated with the aging process. Hardening of the arteries, or *atherosclerosis*, is when the blood vessels that carry oxygenated blood to our organs and other body tissues become clogged with cholesterol and fat, making them more narrow, rigid, and inefficient. When this occurs in the cardiac arteries, it can result in a heart attack. Likewise, our joints become more dehydrated and lose their flexibility as we age. Years of "wear and tear" gradually breakdown the smooth cartilage that coats the surface of our bones causing a condition known as *osteoarthritis* (OA). Healthy articular cartilage is smoother than ice, but as it becomes dried out and brittle, its roughed surface creates friction when the joint moves, and pain results. People with painful joints are less willing to move them which causes the surrounding soft tissue to tighten as well. This creates a vicious cycle that results in greater stiffness.

It is not surprising that the Bible often uses anatomical terms like "stiff-necked" and "hard-hearted" to describe man's perpetually stubborn behavior. Although modern medicine can now graft new vessels to bypass clogged arteries and replace worn out joints with metal and plastic ones, no surgery can fix our stubborn behavior. Just as hardened arteries and stiff joints cause bodily dysfunction, stubbornness can cause dysfunctional relationships with other people as well as with God. The only cure is to replace our stubbornness with love and compassion, and the only physician that can give us that kind of transplant is the divine one that dwells in Heaven. So when we find ourselves experiencing a bad case of stubbornness, we need to seek His intervention – it will make us healthier in both body and spirit!

But our ancestors were proud and stubborn [stiff-necked] and did not obey your commands. They refused to listen; they forgot the miracles you did for them. So they became stubborn and turned against you, choosing a leader to take them back to slavery. But you are a forgiving God. You are kind and full of mercy. You do not become angry quickly, and you have great love. So you did not leave them (Nehemiah 9:16-17).

22

Amazing Capacity

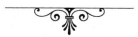

We often refer to a particularly muscular individual as someone who is "built very solid." But in reality, his or her body is still primarily fluid given that approximately 60% of the body's composition is water. In fact, muscle contains 3 to 4 times more water than protein, so a body builder might not be as solid as one would think. About 2/3 of the body's water is contained within its cells. For example, all of our vital organs contain large amounts of water (65-85%) including our heart, lungs, liver, kidneys, and brain. Even our bones are more than 30% water! The remaining 1/3 of our body fluids are found in what we call our extracellular space which includes blood, lymph, spinal fluid, saliva, ocular fluid, the synovial fluid around our joints and tendons, and of course, the excess water we excrete as urine.

The bladder serves as a reservoir for excess fluid and has a maximum capacity of about one liter of urine. This filtered urine drains into the bladder from the kidneys above via the ureters. The middle layer of the bladder wall contains the *detrusor muscle* whose job is to tighten the wall of the bladder and force the urine out through the urethra at its base. In fact, the word detrusor literally means "to thrust out." But the action of the detrusor muscle is not under voluntary control. Instead, stretch receptors in the bladder wall signal the detrusor to contract when the bladder begins to get distended with fluid. This familiar sensation is when we first develop the "urge to go." The scientific term for this automatic response is the *micturition reflex*. As our nervous system matures, we develop the ability to override primitive reflexes, including micturition. So when our circumstances are not ideal for urinating, we can consciously activate the external sphincter which surrounds the urethra and momentarily relax the contracting detrusor. Nevertheless, every reservoir has a maximum capacity and the bladder is no exception. When it reaches its limit, this voluntary control mechanism no longer works and we begin to urinate, ready or not! Anyone who has experienced this embarrassing event realizes that trying to suppress the urge of an expanding bladder too long only creates a bigger problem. Most of us also fail to realize that this same concept applies to stress management. Instead of developing a plan to relieve our daily stresses, we allow them to accumulate like the urine in our bladders until things eventually "spill over," despite our best effort to control them. Then we have a different kind of mess to clean up! Obviously, it would be better to recognize our limits and engage in routine activities such as reading, exercise, tai chi, yoga, meditation or prayer, to void that stress a little at a time. After all, none of us are as solid as we think we are.

> *So I tell you, don't worry about the food or drink you need to live, or about the clothes you need for your body. Life is more than food, and the body is more than clothes. Look at the birds in the air. They don't plant or harvest or store food in barns, but your heavenly Father feeds them. And you know that you are worth much more than the birds. You cannot add any time to your life by worrying about it. And why do you worry about clothes? Look at how the lilies in the field grow. They don't work or make clothes for themselves. But I tell you that even Solomon with his riches was not dressed as beautifully as one of these flowers. God clothes the grass in the field, which is alive today but tomorrow is thrown into the fire. So you can be even more sure that God will clothe you. Don't have so little faith! Don't worry and say, 'What will we eat?' or 'What will we drink?' or 'What will we wear?' The people who don't know God keep trying to get these things, and your Father in heaven knows you need them. Seek first God's kingdom and what God wants. Then all your other needs will be met as well (Matthew 6:25-33).*

23

Amazing Durability

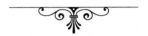

*T*he Gospel of Luke provides a more detailed description than the other three Gospel writers about Christ's physical condition near the end of His life. Most likely this is because Luke was also a physician. The first account we have of Christ's physical suffering refers to His sweat. Luke 22:44 tells us, *"And being in anguish, he prayed more earnestly, and his sweat was like drops of blood falling to the ground."* Whether Luke meant that Jesus' drops of sweat were as large as drops of blood, or whether His sweat actually contained blood, is a source of theological debate. Some scholars claim that sweating blood is impossible. Although it is rare, a condition known as *hematidrosis* can occur when a person is under great emotional stress. In this scenario, tiny capillaries that surround the sweat glands can break, allowing some blood to mix with the sweat. The result is, sweating blood!

Hopefully, none of us will ever have to endure the type of anguish Christ suffered on the cross. Though we may sweat through a lot of stressful circumstances in our lives, we can overcome anything, because His love is greater than any hardship or affliction we may experience.

Love patiently accepts all things. It always trusts, always hopes, and always endures (1 Corinthians 13:7).

24

Amazing Multiplicity

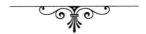

ost body organs have a specialized function; the heart pumps blood, the stomach processes food, the lungs filter air, and so forth. But the liver – now there's a real multi-tasker! Some sources claim that the liver, the largest of our internal organs, can simultaneously perform more than 500 different functions. Basically, it serves as an energy generator, storage facility, and detox center, all in one convenient location. As blood passes from the small intestine into the liver, it removes nutrients and converts them to usable forms of energy to fuel the work of other body organs and tissues. In addition, the liver produces and stores essential vitamins, minerals, and glucose to meet our future energy demands. Finally, it filters a variety of toxic substances from the blood and sends them down the intestinal tract to be discarded as waste products. If the liver failed to perform any of its multiple tasks, our life would end rather abruptly.

Liver disease is caused by a number of factors, but the leading culprits include hepatitis, obesity, cancer, chronic alcohol abuse, and drug toxicity, especially overuse of acetaminophen. *Cirrhosis* is irreversible fibrotic scarring in the liver that occurs in the late stage of hepatic (liver) disease. Although liver transplants are usually successful, hundreds of people die each year waiting for donors. Fortunately, liver tissue can be transplanted from living donors without jeopardizing the health of the "liver giver," because this organ also has the unique ability to regenerate. Interestingly, this characteristic is the focus of a story in Greek mythology involving the Titan Prometheus and his battle with the god, Zeus:

"Having punished mankind, Zeus determined to execute vengeance on Prometheus. He accordingly chained him to a rock in Mount Caucasus, and sent an eagle every day to gnaw away his liver, which grew again every night ready for fresh torments. For thirty years Prometheus endured this fearful punishment; but at length Zeus relented, and permitted his son Heracles (Hercules) to kill the eagle, and the sufferer was released."

In the original text of this story, the liver is referred to as "immortal" which implies that the ancient Greeks knew something about liver's regenerative ability. And yet, reality tells us that no body part is truly immortal as is evidenced by the nearly 15,000 people who die each year from liver disease. Thus, one of our most important jobs is to model and promote healthy life-style habits for the people we work with. Although none of us has a perfect body, the Apostle Paul reminds us that we should honor God with the one we have by taking care of it.

You should know that your body is a temple for the Holy Spirit who is in you. You have received the Holy Spirit from God. So you do not belong to yourselves, because you were bought by God for a price. So honor God with your bodies (1 Corinthians 6:19-20).

25

Amazing Chemistry

Reader's Digest offers suggestions for coping with 13 of the most embarrassing things about our body. Any guess as to what made the list? Most included extra, unwanted things our body sometimes produces such as dandruff, boils, warts, cold sores, leaky urine, and hair that grows in unwanted places like our nose or toes. A few items on the list involved things we may lose as our body ages like a sharp memory or full head of hair. And then there are a number of items that seem to focus on "smelly problems" such as bad breath, perspiration odor, stinky feet, and belching. However, of all the embarrassing things that our body can produce, lose, or do, the passing of intestinal gas, commonly referred to as "farting," may be the most common. The medical term for this physiological event is *flatulence*, and it occurs about 14 to 20 times a day in the average person. Basically, flatulence is caused by trapped air that we probably swallow when we eat and drink, which is one good reason for doing those things more slowly. The sound produced by flatulence is created by vibrations of the rectum when the gas escapes through the anus. The loudness may vary depending on how much pressure is behind the gas, as well as the tightness of the sphincter muscles. Typically, flatulence is more likely to occur during sleep when the sphincter is relaxed. It is also caused by the bacterial fermentation of undigested food, particularly carbohydrates that are moving through the intestines. A typical *flatus* (medical term for a fart) is composed of about 59% nitrogen, 21% hydrogen, 9% carbon dioxide, 7% methane, 4% oxygen, and a small amount of hydrogen sulfide gas. It is the sulfur in that last component which creates the bad odor and makes flatulence so offensive that it can sometimes clear a room! The more sulfur-rich our diet is, the more terrible our flatulence will smell. Some foods contain more sulfur than others, especially eggs and high-fiber foods such as beans, peas, cabbage, root vegetables and many types of fruits. However, these fiber-rich foods have other nutritional value, so we don't want to completely eliminate them from our diet.

Besides the embarrassing sound and unpleasant odor associated with flatulence, it also has some inherent dangers. The methane and hydrogen in bacteria-produced flatus can make our gas highly flammable. In rare cases, a build-up of flammable gasses in the intestines has caused explosions during intestinal surgeries! Furthermore, some people suggest that global warming may be partially attributed to the emission of methane, a "greenhouse gas," produced by animals which consume large quantities of fiber such as livestock and the tiny, wood-munching termite. According to the Environmental Protection Agency, enteric fermentation (animal flatulence) produces 25% of the methane emissions in the U.S. That is roughly equivalent to the amount produced by natural gas and petroleum industry!

So how do we deal with this embarrassing body function? Most people try to inhibit flatulence when in public situations. However suppression of this release of gas is likely to cause greater discomfort than the social embarrassment. Maybe we should just accept flatulence as God's occasional reminder that we are all human beings who tend to create "a little stink" in each other's lives, no matter how hard we try to avoid it. So whenever we pass a little more intestinal gas, it should remind us to pass a little less judgment on those whose imperfections tend to offend us from time to time.

We all make many mistakes. If people never said anything wrong, they would be perfect and able to control their entire selves, too (James 3:2).

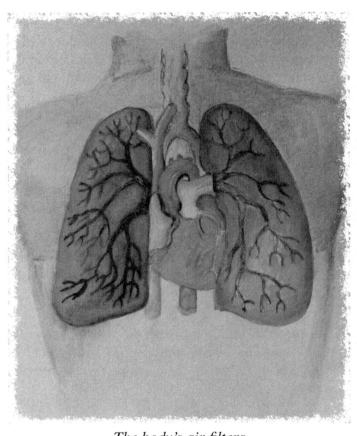

The body's air filters

26

Amazing Vitality

*R*espiration is an act that all living creatures take for granted even though we do it about 22,000 times a day. As the air enters our lungs through two large tubes, or *bronchi*, it is channeled down through one of the multiple lobes and segments of lung tissue by way of smaller airways known as bronchioles. Finally, the air reaches the functional units of the lung, the *alveoli*, which resemble tiny clusters of grapes. Each day more than 40 billion trillion molecules of oxygen are absorbed through 480 million alveoli whose combined surface area is roughly the size of a tennis court. This vital oxygen is then infused into the 2400 gallons or so of blood that is subsequently pumped through the heart and delivered to the rest of the body. And this cycle continues on a 24/7 basis without any conscious effort. If we had to focus on the complexities of this physiological process, no doubt there would be little time to think about anything else! Although the lungs are the primary organs for respiration, variations in our breathing rate and pattern are controlled by neural structures found in the base of the brain (i.e., the brainstem). These control centers respond to chemical signals from major arteries that detect fluctuations in the levels of oxygen and carbon dioxide in our blood. Thus, they can tell the lungs to increase or decrease the respiratory rate as needed to meet the changing demands of our activity level and maintain our vitality.

Throughout the Bible, living creatures are described as those who have the "breath of life." Even though we now define clinical death by the cessation of a heart beat as well as respiration, the Bible consistently describes death as a time when someone has "breathed his [or her] last." Thus, the act of respiration is intimately associated with life itself. Does that mean that people who can no longer breathe on their own and require the assistance of a mechanical ventilator are actually dead? That question becomes more than a physiological issue, and is the subject of continuous debate among medical ethicists. Regardless of one's beliefs regarding end-of-life care, we should probably all heed the message in the famous quote, *"Life is not measured by the number of breaths we take, but by the moments that take our breath away."* Although there is no agreement regarding the original author of this quote, its implication is clear – we should focus more on the intangible things that enhance the meaning and quality of our lives, than the physiological measures which quantify it. So take a moment to deeply inhale the breath of life and remember to thank our Creator for this precious gift.

> *Then the Lord God took dust from the ground and formed a man from it. He breathed the breath of life into the man's nose, and the man became a living person (Genesis 2:7).*

27

Amazing Continuity

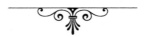

*O*ne of the most unique muscles in our body is the *diaphragm* – it controls our every breath! This dome-shaped muscle forms the floor of the thoracic cavity and the ceiling of the abdominal cavity with multiple openings, or hiatuses, that provide passage for the esophagus, major blood vessels, and nerves between the two segments of the trunk. Peripherally it attaches to the cartilage of the lower six ribs as well as the tip of the sternum (xiphoid process) and anterior aspect of the first three lumbar vertebrae and their disks. Its fibers unite to form a central tendon which attaches to the inferior aspect of the pericardium, the sac of fibrous tissue which surrounds the heart. Thus, when this muscle contracts it acts like a bellows by pulling the thorax downward, creating a negative pressure which facilitates the flow of air into the lungs. Relaxation of the diaphragm allows it to retract upward again which passively assists with expiration. Although other muscles may produce far greater strength and power, the diaphragm has little competition when it comes to endurance. It contracts continuously, about 22,000 times a day, without stopping. But occasionally its smooth rhythm gets interrupted by an involuntary spasm known *as synchronous diaphragmatic flutter* (SDF), or *singultus*. Sounds pretty serious, doesn't it? But anyone who has experienced the hiccups knows that this is usually a rather benign and temporary affliction.

Several things are believed to trigger an episode of hiccups such as gulping food down too quickly, drinking something much hotter or colder than the stomach's temperature, or experiencing some emotional shock. However, none of these factors were responsible for the record-setting case of singultus that an Iowa man named Charles Osborne laid claim to. His hiccups began on June 5, 1922, when he was hanging a 350 pound hog that he was preparing to butcher. And they persisted for the next 68 years despite trying every known cure! Osborne's doctors later concluded that his case was probably caused by the rupture of a tiny blood vessel in that portion of his midbrain which normally inhibits the hiccup response. Although Osborne initially hiccupped around 40 times a minute, the rate slowed as he aged and mysteriously stopped about a year prior to his death.

Experts estimated that Osborne hiccupped over 430 million times during his 97-year lifetime, but he did not let these little interruptions stop him from leading a fairly normal life. Likewise, when life takes an unexpected turn, we can't let those "hiccups" deter us. Certainly Moses encountered his share of hiccups when he was leading the Israelites to the Promised Land, but he persevered. And if you're a health care professional, you are probably treating people with lots of different hiccups, not to mention some of your own. Fortunately, most of life's hiccups are more of an inconvenience than a serious problem, and many of them teach us valuable lessons, offer unexpected opportunities, or make us more resilient. So maybe we should learn to take them in stride like Charles Osborne did. After all, just because our diaphragm may hiccup once in a while, that doesn't mean we're going to stop breathing.

Do not worry about anything, but pray and ask God for everything you need, always giving thanks. And God's peace, which is so great we cannot understand it, will keep your hearts and minds in Christ Jesus (Philippians 4:6-7).

28

Amazing Recovery

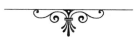

*H*ow many times have you pandiculated today? Chances are you were either bored or sleepy when you did it. *Pandiculation* is actually the medical term for the combined yawning and stretching that occurs when we feel drowsy. It is a physiological process that we share with all other animals including fish and reptiles. However, the reason for yawning is not clearly understood. Many believe it is the body's way of increasing the intake of oxygen to the brain when our level of alertness begins to decline. It is similar to blowing air on burning embers to help rekindle a fire. Others contend that yawning rejuvenates us because it provides a mechanism to rid our body of excess carbon dioxide that builds up in our blood. Thus, a good yawn and stretch can help improve circulation. Interestingly, people who are severely ill or psychotic rarely yawn. So when we see a seriously ill patient begin to yawn again, we should recognize this as one of the earliest signs of recovery. And when we feel the urge to pandiculate, we should consider it God's way of revitalizing our mind, body, and spirit. With that renewed energy, we can better pursue our purpose in life and, hopefully, help others who are trying to pursue theirs.

Even children become tired and need to rest, and young people trip and fall. But the people who trust the Lord will become strong again. They will rise up as an eagle in the sky; they will run and not need rest; they will walk and not become tired (Isaiah 40:30-31).

29

Amazing Barbarity

*A*lthough there are many physiological factors that may be postulated to contribute to death during a crucifixion, asphyxia (suffocation from lack of oxygen) is believed to be the primary cause. As mentioned previously, normal inhalation occurs when the diaphragm contracts to create a negative pressure that allows air to flow into the lungs. This movement can be facilitated by the intercostal muscles that are located between each rib. These muscles, assisted by muscles of the shoulder girdle, help expand the rib cage and elevate the chest. Exhalation is normally a relatively passive movement caused by relaxation of these muscles of inspiration. However, during a crucifixion, the fixed, outstretched position of the victim's shoulders and arms prevents further expansion of the chest wall. In addition, the weight of the hanging body stretches the chest vertically, thereby inhibiting the process of exhalation. Thus, breathing is shallow at best, and insufficient to support life, particularly in such a painful and stressed physiological state. As a result, there is a build-up of carbon dioxide (*hypercarbia*) which causes a slow suffocation. Victims struggle to push and pull the rib cage up with their nailed feet and hands to assist with the act of exhalation. History tells us that past executioners often forcibly fractured the victim's legs (i.e., *crucifracture*) to prevent this biomechanical assistance and hasten death. Certainly it is easy to understand the significance of the term "excruciating pain" that derives its meaning from the Latin word "excruciatus" which literally means "out of the cross." However, only by understanding the true nature of human pain and suffering, are we able to develop compassion and empathy for those who need our help.

> *Praise be to the God and Father of our Lord Jesus Christ. God is the Father who is full of mercy and all comfort. He comforts us every time we have trouble, so when others have trouble, we can comfort them with the same comfort God gives us. We share in the many sufferings of Christ. In the same way, much comfort comes to us through Christ. If we have troubles, it is for your comfort and salvation, and if we have comfort, you also have comfort. This helps you to accept patiently the same sufferings we have (2 Corinthians 1:3-6).*

30

Amazing Tranquility

A person can live about 40 days without food, about 7 days without water, and about 6 to 8 minutes without air. Those facts are not too startling. However, another physiological function that is vital to our survival is sleep. Humans can actually survive longer without food than without sleep. After a few sleepless nights, a person is likely to start experiencing radical personality and psychological changes, a phenomenon that has been demonstrated in several scientific experiments and reports of military personnel or psychiatric patients who have gone without sleep for more than a day or two. In many cases, this sleep deprivation ultimately results in suicide.

Those unlucky individuals who inherit a rare disorder known as *Fatal Familial Insomnia* (FFI) usually die within two years from lack of sleep. FFI has no known cure and involves progressively worsening insomnia which leads to hallucinations, delirium, and confusion that mimics dementia. This disorder is probably misnamed because death actually results from multiple organ failure rather than sleep deprivation. The pathological processes include degeneration of the thalamus and other areas of the brain, an overactive sympathetic nervous system, hypertension, fever, tremors, stupor, weight loss, and disruption of the body's endocrine system. FFI has been diagnosed in less than 40 families worldwide, including Chicago music teacher, Michael Corke, who was featured in the BBC documentary, *The Man Who Never Slept*. Thus, the next time you feel yourself nodding off, just remember that the ability to sleep is truly a life-sustaining blessing. And as the Psalmist tells us, the tranquility of sleep is a gift that symbolizes God's love.

> *If the Lord doesn't build the house, the builders are working for nothing. If the Lord doesn't guard the city, the guards are watching for nothing. It is no use for you to get up early and stay up late, working for a living. The Lord gives sleep to those he loves (Psalm 127:1-2).*

31

Amazing Imagery

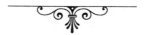

*H*ave you ever tried to tell someone about a dream only to discover that you cannot recall most of it? Most people dream a couple hours a night and usually have multiple dreams. However, half of what we dream about is forgotten within 5 minutes of awakening, and within 10 minutes, 90% of dreams are lost. According to surveys, the five most common dreams involve falling, being pursued or attacked, trying to perform a task repeatedly and failing, work or school activities, and sexual experiences. Most people believe that dreams are just symbolic representations of thoughts or ideas that the unconscious brain is trying to connect. Some of the most important inventions and discoveries were inspired by dreams. Examples of creative dreamers include Dimitri Medeleyev who developed the periodic table of elements, James Watson who discovered DNA's double helix structure, Elias Howe who invented the sewing machine, Tesla's creation of the alternating current generator, and Larry Page's idea for Google. Others believe that dreams serve as warnings for potential life-threatening events. Abraham Lincoln had multiple dreams predicting his own assassination. Many of the 9/11 victims had premonitions of an impending disaster, as did several passengers on the *Titanic* and a few fortunate souls who heeded the warning and decided not to board the ship. Even the famous psychologist, Carl Jung, who routinely analyzed and interpreted the dreams of others, had a foreboding dream of his own in June of 1914. Jung saw a massive sea turned to blood and filled with drowning bodies, followed by a cold wave that froze the entire country. Just a few weeks later, Jung witnessed the outbreak of World War I.

Of course, another popular notion about the purpose of dreams is that they provide a mechanism for God to communicate with people. Interestingly, dreams are mentioned 224 times in the scriptures, and nearly 1/3 of the content in the Bible refers to dreams and visions of important people such as Abraham, Joseph, Daniel, Ezekiel, Joseph (Jesus' father), Mary (Jesus' mother), Paul, Cornelius, John, and others. Obviously when the message is worth remembering, God will find a way to override our brain's physiologic tendency to forget!

The Lord answered me: 'Write down the vision; write it clearly on clay tablets so whoever reads it can run to tell others. It is not yet time for the message to come true, but that time is coming soon; the message will come true' *(Habakkuk 2:2-3).*

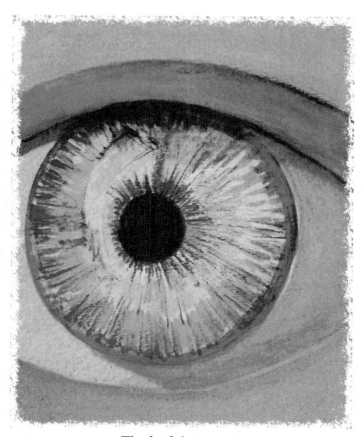

The body's camera

32

Amazing Acuity

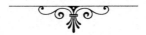

*D*id you know that 80% of the things we learn and remember are determined by what we see? So our vision obviously plays an extremely important role in our brain's development. Because the eye has more than 2 million working parts, some sources claim its complexity is second only to that of the brain. The external surface of the eyeball actually constitutes only 1/6 of its total structure. The portion of the eye that determines one's eye color is the iris. The pupil is the black dot (actually a hole) in the center of the iris, and the white surrounding is the sclera. These parts are protected by a transparent cover called the cornea which is comparable to the lens of a camera. Once the cornea focuses the light, the iris adjusts the size of the pupil to regulate the amount of light needed to visualize the image. In this way, the iris functions much like the aperture of a camera. Once the visual image is projected through the pupil it encounters the lens of the eye which refines the focus of the light before projecting the image onto the retina behind it. The retina contains two types of photoreceptors, *rods* and *cones*. The rods are more numerous (approximately 120 million of them!) and more sensitive than the cones in giving our visual images their clear resolution. However, it is the cones in the retina that enable us to see color. These 6 to 7 million cones are most densely concentrated in a central yellow portion of the retina known as the *macula*. This is why people who experience macular degeneration tend to lose their central vision and much of their color sensitivity. Together the cones and rods convert our visual images into precise electrical signals which are sent via the optic nerve to the visual cortex of the brain for interpretation. The dual input from both eyes contributes to our ability to construct 3-dimensional images of our surroundings and gives us the depth perception needed to move about safely in our environment. In addition, the tiny muscles of the eye allow us to visually track objects in our environment without constantly turning our head. This mobile function of the eye keeps us oriented in space and is critical to the maintenance of balance.

Aside from the marvelous acuity provided by these anatomic cameras, we often hear the eyes referred to as the "windows of the soul." Perhaps this relates to our ability to detect something about an individual's emotional state when we look into his or her eyes. Wide-open eyes may portray fear, anxiety, or arousal, while squinting eyes suggest disapproval, suspicion, or disgust. Darting eyes indicate one's nervousness or insecurity, and tightly closed eyes suggest an impending threat. Moist eyes are commonly associated with sadness (unless we're dicing onions), and "dreamy" eyes are a sure sign that love is in the air! Some people even claim that quick eye movements to the left indicate when a person is telling the truth versus movements to the right which might suggest that person is lying. Quite often, we may find that these emotions provide the key to their understanding a patient's physical symptoms. So the next time we want to understand someone's physical problem, we should try to be more than just a good listener. By making good eye contact, we might just discover a diagnostic clue that the rest of the body was not willing or able to reveal.

> *Your eye is a light for the body. When your eyes are good, your whole body will be full of light. But when your eyes are evil, your whole body will be full of darkness. So be careful not to let the light in you become darkness. If your whole body is full of light, and none of it is dark, then you will shine bright, as when a lamp shines on you (Luke 11:34-36).*

33

Amazing Complexity

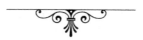

*C*ertainly most of us value our eyesight as one of our most critical and complex senses. Although many individuals can learn to function independently without sight, most of us would be rendered helpless by a sudden onset of blindness. So it's nice to know that our body has some built-in protection for our eyes. For example, eyelashes help to keep dirt out of our eyes and eyebrows help prevent sweat from running into them. Tears are like natural eye drops that keep our eyes clean and moist. Regular blinking helps wash these tears over our eyeballs. Like most reflexes, *blinking* is a protective mechanism that shields the eye from trauma whenever an object threatens to strike its surface. This reflex is actually an extremely complex interaction among multiple ocular muscles that operate synergistically via parallel circuits in the brain stem in as little as 3/10 of a second! Although estimates vary, most sources claim that the average human blinks about 15 to 20 times a minute. That adds up to approximately 28,000 times a day and over 10 million times each year. If we were to save all the times our eyes blink in the average lifetime and use them all at once we would see nothing but darkness for over a year! Because blinking is known to be one of the fastest reflexes in the human body, the Apostle Paul uses this analogy to convey just how quickly our lives will be transformed when the promise of Christ's return is fulfilled.

But look! I tell you this secret: We will not all sleep in death, but we will all be changed. It will take only a second—as quickly as an eye blinks—when the last trumpet sounds. The trumpet will sound, and those who have died will be raised to live forever, and we will all be changed (1 Corinthians 15:51-52).

34

Amazing Perceptivity

*E*mbedded deep within the center of our brain is a pea-sized structure whose name reveals its unique pine cone shape – the *pineal gland* (or pineal body). Throughout history, the pine cone has symbolized human enlightenment which gives us some insight into both the real and speculated functions of this tiny gland. Although it secretes many different hormones, the pineal gland is the primary manufacturer of *melatonin* which helps regulate our circadian rhythm. It is believed that photoreceptors contained in the pineal gland respond to light, thereby causing it to secrete more melatonin when our environment is dark (to lull us to sleep) and suppress its production during daylight hours (to keep us awake). This response to changing light conditions may be one reason the pineal gland has been nicknamed "the third eye." Among its other unique aspects, this endocrine gland is noted for being the first to form in the developing fetus at 3 weeks of age, having a blood supply that is only exceeded by the kidneys, and producing calcified particles known as "brain sand" as we age.

Because the true physiological functions of the pineal gland were not discovered until the 1960s, it has been the object of speculation related to its mystical and spiritual power for many centuries. Three hundred years before the birth of Christ, the Greek physician, Herophilus, noted the unique anatomical configuration of the pineal gland and concluded that it must play a major role in our consciousness. In 1662, French mathematician and philosopher, René Descartes, popularized another nickname for the pineal gland when he declared it to be the "seat of the soul." Descartes' obsession with finding a literal connection between the body and the soul led him to make many erroneous assumptions about the pineal gland's structure and function. Despite our current knowledge of its true anatomical and physiological nature, many of these speculations continue as various new age spiritualists claim that the pineal gland secretes natural psychedelic substances, similar to LSD, which telepathically link our earthly consciousness to the spiritual realm. This speculation has been used to explain the vivid visual nature of some dreams as well as the realistic out-of-body experiences reported by many people who have had close encounters with death. But whether or not one chooses to believe that the pineal gland plays a direct role in our connection with God, there's no denying that He can and will find a way to communicate with us when He needs to.

God does speak—sometimes one way and sometimes another—even though people may not understand it. He speaks in a dream or a vision of the night when people are in a deep sleep, lying on their beds. He speaks in their ears and frightens them with warnings to turn them away from doing wrong and to keep them from being proud (Job 33:14-17).

35

Amazing Excitability

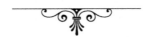

*T*he brain is a marvelous, intricate network of nerve cells, or *neurons*, that literally regulate the function of every other part of the body. The brain sends its messages back and forth by way of electrical impulses that are transmitted through this vast neural network. Although these neurons provide the highways for these impulses to travel on, they cannot actually deliver the message without a little help. When the nerve reaches its target tissue or organ, it must release chemicals known as *neurotransmitters* which deliver the brain's message across the gap between the nerve ending and the target tissue/organ. Basically, they function like tiny ferry boats, only much faster!

A German scientist named Otto Loewi was the first to discover this chemical mechanism for transmitting nerve impulses in 1921. He submerged two frog hearts in connected containers filled with saline solution. After stimulating the vagus nerve to slow the pulse rate of the first frog heart, Loewi observed a similar slowing in the rate of the second frog heart caused by a substance that was flowing from one heart to the other. This substance was later identified as the neurotransmitter, acetylcholine, which is involved with the transmission of motor impulses. Like acetylcholine, some neurotransmitters serve an excitatory function as they help activate or speed up certain bodily functions like our breathing, heart rate, or digestive process. Epinephrine, also known as adrenaline, is a good example of an excitatory neurotransmitter. Many people have experienced an "adrenaline rush" that is actually a release of this stress hormone which enables the body to react to urgent situations by temporarily increasing our heart rate, respiratory rate, and blood pressure. Other excitatory neurotransmitters such as dopamine are responsible for helping us focus our attention, stay on task, and remain motivated when we have a complex mental task to complete. We also have inhibitory neurotransmitters that are released when we need to slow down or block certain bodily functions. For example, serotonin is an inhibitory neurotransmitter that helps maintain our mental balance by preventing overstimulation of our brain, similar to the effect of valium.

Unfortunately, our bodies can sometimes run low on neurotransmitters which may reduce our ability to perform certain mental or physical activities or control undesired reactions such as anxiety, pain, and depression. One source estimates that as many as 86% of Americans have suboptimal neurotransmitter levels caused by factors such as stress, poor diet, drugs, alcohol, caffeine, toxic chemicals in the environment, and genetic predisposition. The cumulative effect of these factors can ultimately damage our immune system. The neuromuscular disease, myasthenia gravis (MG), is a prime example. In MG, the immune system seems to produce certain antibodies that block or destroy the receptor sites for acetylcholine in the muscle. Without the ability to cross this junction and excite the muscle, there is a rapid onset of muscle fatigue and weakness.

In some ways, we might think of neurotransmitters as the anatomic equivalent of God's grace. As imperfect people, the only way to bridge the gap between ourselves and a perfect God is through the grace He provided with His Son's sacrifice on the cross. That grace facilitates our communication with God. Without this ultimate neurotransmitter, we could never make that connection with our "heavenly brain."

Jesus answered, "I am the way, and the truth, and the life. The only way to the Father is through me (John 14:6).

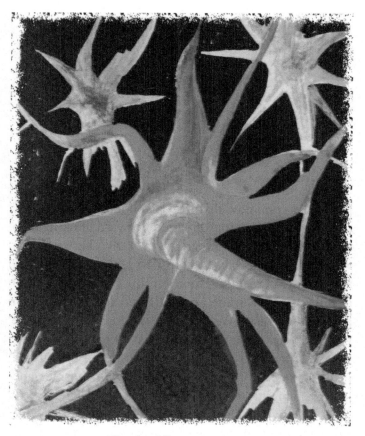

The body's messengers

36

Amazing Reactivity

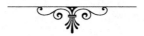

*D*id you know that frogs cannot hop backwards? It's not that they are more forward thinking than the rest of the animal kingdom, but rather because their vestibular system has no ability to sense movement in a backward direction. However, the human vestibular system is much more sophisticated than that of our amphibian cousin. We can sense motion whether we're moving forward, backward, sideways, or vertically. This sensory function, when augmented by our vision and position sensors (*proprioceptors*) in our muscles and joints, enables us to maintain our balance whether we're static or moving. The anatomical apparatus responsible for detecting and reacting to directional movement is known as the *labyrinth*, and we have one located in each inner ear. These structures, a little smaller than the size of a penny, resemble a snail with three circular append-ages on its back. These appendages are fluid-filled canals that are oriented perpendicular to one another. At the base of these canals are bulbous areas called *otoliths* which contain tiny hairs that are anchored to sensory nerves. When the head tilts in one direction, these hairs bend in the opposite direction. Attached to the free ends of these hairs are small calcium crystals called *otoconia,* or "ear rocks," which act as small weights to make the hair movement more pronounced and easier to detect. As we age or experience repetitive head trauma, these otoconia may break loose and find their way into one of the semi-circular canals where they disrupt our equilibrium and cause episodes of dizziness. This condition is known as BPPV which stands for *benign, paroxysmal, positional vertigo.* Although BPPV can be quite disabling, it is easily treated using a variety of head repositioning maneuvers that help move the displaced otoconia back to their "home" in the otoliths. The most common repositioning technique is known as the Epley maneuver which boasts a success rate of at least 80%.

Some of us may feel like an ear rock at times – something shakes our world and throws us off balance. We may feel like we're just spinning in circles. But if we place our trust God, He will reposition us and restore the equilibrium in our lives. And His treatment technique is even simpler than performing an Epley maneuver – all we have to do is kneel down and look up!

But those who follow the true way come to the light, and it shows that the things they do were done through God (John 3:21).

37

Amazing Sensitivity

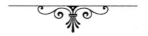

Olfaction, or the act of smelling, is one of our most primitive senses. Every time we inhale, currents of air carry various molecular odorants up through the nostrils to millions of receptor neurons that lie on the surface of the nose. Each of these olfactory neurons contains tiny filaments called cilia which project into the atmosphere and bind with the molecules that contain specific odorants. Each receptor has a binding site that is just the right shape to fit with a specific molecule. The interaction of the right molecule with the right receptor causes that receptor to change its shape and send an electrical signal to the brain which converts the signal into a smell. Although references vary, most suggest that humans can detect somewhere between 20,000 and 50,000 different scents. By comparison, a dog's sniffer is thought to be at least 10,000 times more sensitive than that of us, nasally-challenged humans. The difference in olfactory ability can be attributed to two anatomic variations. First, the internal surface area of a dog's nose is about 60 times larger than ours and contains about 1 billion olfactory receptor cells compared to approximately 12 million in the human nose. And if that dog is a bloodhound, we can magnify the number another four times! Second, the portion of the dog's brain that interprets scents is 40% larger than the same portion of the human brain.

But do dogs remember those scents in the same way that humans do? Because olfaction is handled by the same part of the brain (the limbic system) that handles memories and emotions, certain smells often trigger past memories. While visual images may fade within days, the memory of a smell can persist for many years. For example, the scent of pine may remind us of Christmas or the smell of fresh-baked cookies may take us back to mom's kitchen. Likewise, unpleasant odors may provoke even stronger emotional responses. Interestingly, many passages in the Old Testament tell us that even God was emotionally moved by His sense of smell in response to the people's burnt offerings and sacrifices – further evidence of yet another way in which we are made in His image.

Put all of these in the hands of Aaron and his sons, and tell them to present them as an offering to the Lord. Then take them from their hands and burn them on the altar with the whole burnt offering. This is an offering made by fire to the Lord; its smell is pleasing to the Lord (Exodus 29:24-25).

38

Amazing Purity

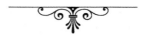

*A*lthough we typically think of the nose as an important sensory organ and filter for the vital air we breathe, did you ever wonder what makes it run? The mucous produced by our nose (almost a liter a day) is normally channeled to the back of the throat where it is swallowed without conscious effort. However, when the nose gets too cold, its blood vessels dilate to increase blood flow and warm the air before it enters the lungs. A side effect of this increased blood flow is the stimulation of glands that produce nasal mucous. Excess mucous that cannot be swallowed tends to simply run out of the nose. A similar response occurs when the nasal cavity is invaded by viruses, germs, or allergens which stimulate these "snot-producing" glands to clear away the offending organism. However, the nose's tendency to run when we cry is simply due to an over-production of tears which drain into our nose and mix with the mucous that is already there. So it seems that our nose can also function as an important escape hatch. These escaping tears not only help wash out our eyes and nose, they also help cleanse our soul. As stated in Psalm 30:5b, *"Weeping may stay for a night, but rejoicing comes in the morning."* Although the nose serves as a useful conduit to rid our body of excess mucous and tears, the Bible reminds us that God has provided an even greater mechanism to purify our hearts and bring us closer to Him.

Let us come near to God with a sincere heart and a sure faith, because we have been made free from a guilty conscience, and our bodies have been washed with pure water (Hebrews 10:22).

39

Amazing Circuitry

*L*ike many body parts, our brains have a right and left side, known as *cerebral hemispheres*, which are connected by a central bundle of nerve fibers called the *corpus callosum*. In general, each side of the brain controls what happens on the opposite side of the body. Thus, someone with a brain injury or stroke in the left cerebral hemisphere is likely to experience some type of sensory, perceptual, or motor deficits on the right side of the body. Although these hemispheres grossly appear alike, their asymmetry is revealed in functional MRI studies which show selective activation of different parts of the brain when people perform various tasks. For example, the left side is activated during speech and language skills, while the right side is more involved with tasks that require focused attention on visual and spatial relationships. The theory of brain *lateralization*, or hemispheric specialization, arose from the Nobel Prize-winning work of psycho-biologist,

Dr. Roger Sperry. His theories helped popularize the notion of right-brain versus left-brain dominance which has been used for years to classify people as logical, analytical "left-brainers" or intuitive, creative "right-brainers." However, recent scientific studies have debunked the left-brain/right-brain myth and shifted our focus to cognitive theories which emphasize variation in how the brain integrates the function of its multiple parts to produce different thinking modes. For example, Dr. Anthony Gregorc identified two dimensions to our thinking process – one based on the quality of our perceptions (concrete vs. abstract) and one based on our ordering ability (sequential vs. random). More recently, Kosslyn and Miller proposed a "top brain, bottom brain" theory to explain how different people process information and make decisions. They contend that top part of the brain is more involved with planning and organization, while the bottom brain pays more attention to what's going on in the environment. Their theory helps explain why some people easily generate new ideas, but it takes other people to figure out how to make those ideas work. It also explains why some people are more spontaneous risk-takers, while others act in a more reserved and deliberate manner.

Finally, neuroimaging studies have also revealed clear differences in the neural connectivity of male and female brains. Men's brains tend to form more intra-hemispheric connections from front to back, which facilitate the coordination of motor activities. In contrast, women's brains usually have a larger corpus callosum due to a greater number of interhemispheric connections which allows them to easily merge their analytical and intuitive processes. Regardless of which explanation makes most sense, our brains are clearly more than just a gelatinous mass of neurons! Because we all develop and use the specialized parts of our brains differently, we should be eager to share our thoughts and ideas with one another. If not, we run the risk of developing a skewed perception of how things are and a very biased view of how things should be. Jesus obviously recognized the benefit of "brain picking" when he chose not one, but twelve, followers. These men came from diverse occupations and social backgrounds, demonstrated contrasting personalities and divergent views, and used different approaches to spread the gospel. But it was through a combined, integrated effort that these apostles were able to fulfill the one purpose to which they were called.

Does your life in Christ give you strength? Does his love comfort you? Do we share together in the spirit? Do you have mercy and kindness? If so, make me very happy by having the same thoughts, sharing the same love, and having one mind and purpose. When you do things, do not let selfishness or pride be your guide. Instead, be humble and give more honor to others than to yourselves (Philippians 2:1-3).

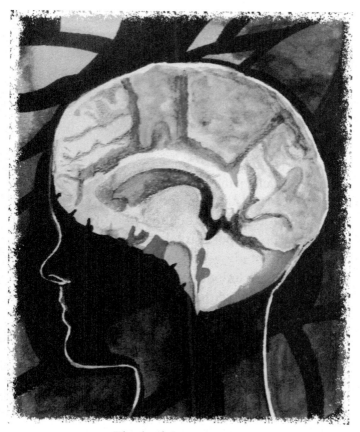

The body's computer

40

Amazing Memory

*A*n article in the January 2007 issue of *Cognition* reported that episodes from our past are remembered faster and better while in a body position similar to the pose struck during the actual event. Although this study generally asked subjects to recall more pleasant or emotionally neutral memories, some practitioners believe the energy associated with traumatic events in our lives is also "remembered" by the body, particularly the *myofascial tissues* (strong connective tissue found between muscles and bones), even though it may be blocked from our consciousness. This theory may explain why the certain myofascial release techniques often trigger an emotional, as well as a physical, response from the patient. This notion of body memory also helps explain phenomena such as phantom sensations in people who have had limbs amputated or phobic reactions to certain environmental stimuli such as heights or enclosed spaces.

Evidently our brain is not the only body part capable of storing emotional memories.

A more recent study published by Dias and Ressler in *Nature Neuroscience* speculates that some of our memories may actually be inherited. These researchers found that laboratory mice which received an electric shock when exposed to the smell of acetophenone (a chemical scent similar to that of cherries and almonds) eventually shuddered in fear when exposed to the scent even in the absence of the electric shock. More interesting was the fact that the first- and second-generation offspring of these mice demonstrated the same adverse reaction to acetophenone even though they had neither been previously exposed to the scent nor the noxious stimulus associated with it. Similar reports by Paul Pearsall and others indicate that many organ transplant recipients, particularly heart transplants, have a tendency to inherit some of the memories, talents, or personality traits which their deceased donors possessed. These stories have caused some scientists to speculate on the possibility of "cellular memory." Obviously we cannot always determine the source of our memories, good or bad, nor can we necessarily understand their significance. But we do know that God created memories for a reason, and in most cases, He intended for these memories to protect us from future harm.

But be careful! Watch out and don't forget the things you have seen. Don't forget them as long as you live, but teach them to your children and grandchildren (Deuteronomy 4:9).

41

Amazing Senility

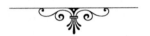

*O*bviously God gave us memories for several good reasons – to help shape our personalities, build meaningful relationships, teach us valuable lessons, and so forth. In fact, most of our strongest emotional responses are tied to either a pleasant or unpleasant memory. So what happens when someone loses those memories? Are they still the same person? Typically memory loss is associated with some type of brain damage. Stories of individuals who exhibit temporary or permanent amnesia following a head injury are not uncommon, and many have become the storyline for popular movies such as *The Bourne Identity, Total Recall, Regarding Henry,* and *The Long Kiss Goodnight.* But, by far, the most devastating type of memory loss is that associated with various types of dementia such as Alzheimer's disease (AD). AD not only robs its victims of their memories, it can eventually destroy their ability to perform the most basic human functions such as eating, speaking, and moving. Deposits of sticky protein material known as amyloid plaques, coupled with tangled nerve fibers, literally "short circuit" the brain's neural network. Familiar possessions are seen as foreign objects, and loved ones become strangers. As neural connections gradually disappear, the brain is like a computer disk that has been erased. Although some information may still be stored there, it can no longer be retrieved. The person with dementia eventually loses his or her identity and withdraws from the world like an infant returning to the womb. Thus, the phrase *"Once an adult, twice a child"* is commonly used to describe the progressive nature of AD.

Despite this dismal prognosis, scientists continue to unravel the mysteries of AD and discover factors that may help protect us from the consequences of this dreaded disease. In his famous "Nun Study," Dr. David Snowdon was among the first to document the benefits of mental exercise in reducing the risk of AD. This longitudinal study began in 1986 and focused on a group of 678 retired nuns from the School Sisters of Notre Dame who led a relatively healthy and homogenous lifestyle. Among the most intriguing of Snowdon's findings was the linguistic analysis he performed on biographical essays written by these nuns when they were young women. Those who wrote more complex sentences, used richer vocabulary, and expressed more positive emotions were far less likely to develop dementia later in life than those whose writing was more simplistic or negative. Following their deaths, autopsies performed on the brains of these nuns often revealed pathological evidence of advanced AD even though they exhibited no outward signs of the disease when they were living. Several recent research studies have supported Snowdon's deduction that both mental and physical activities may have a protective effect on brain health. Thus, it seems the best way to help our patients preserve their memories is to encourage them to "train their brain" and "hustle their muscle!"

You know these things, and you are very strong in the truth, but I will always help you remember them. I think it is right for me to help you remember as long as I am in this body. I know I must soon leave this body, as our Lord Jesus Christ has shown me. I will try my best so that you may be able to remember these things even after I am gone (2 Peter 1:12-15).

42

Amazing Connectivity

everal years ago, a story about *laminin* began circulating around the internet. Laminins are extracellular proteins that have three short arms and one longer arm. These arms are like sticky tentacles that enable these proteins to attach to each other and form a foundational structure called a *basement membrane*. Because this membrane's function is to hold all the cells of that tissue together, some references describe laminins as a sort of cellular "scaffolding" or "glue" that is vital to the survival of all our body's tissues. When laminins become defective, they cause pathological changes within the tissue as noted in some types of muscular dystrophy and cancer.

Regardless of its important function, what really captured the attention

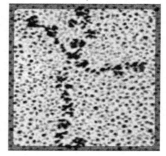

of so many people was the release of photographs taken with an electron microscope which revealed the cross-shaped configuration of laminins. The unique molecular arrangement of these proteins has led some popular evangelists to describe them as the "cross within us." Whether these protein molecules truly resemble a cross or not, the adhesive function of laminins should always remind us of the tremendous sacrifice that Jesus made to cement the bond between God and man.

> *Speaking the truth with love, we will grow up in every way into Christ, who is the head. The whole body depends on Christ, and all the parts of the body are joined and held together. Each part does its own work to make the whole body grow and be strong with love (Ephesians 4:15-16).*

43

Amazing Synergy

*H*uman hair fibers are protein filaments that emerge from follicles found in the skin (i.e., dermis). The living part of the hair is anchored in the follicle, and approximately 70 grams of force is required to dislodge it. The number of hair follicles on our head varies by hair color. Blondes have the most, averaging 120,000 to 140,000. People with dark hair (black or brown) have approximately 100,000 to 110,000 follicles, and redheads have the least with only about 86,000 to 90,000. Regardless of how many we start with, most people lose between 50 and 100 hairs a day unless some pathological condition accelerates that loss. With the exception of bone marrow, hair reproduces and grows faster than any tissue in the human body. During our lifetime, each hair follicle will produce about 20 to 30 hairs which can last anywhere from 2 to 7 years each. Fortunately, most people have about 100,000 hair follicles, so there are plenty to spare!

One human hair can support 3.5 ounces of force – that's about the weight of two full size candy bars. The ultimate strength of hair is about 380 MPa (1 MPa = 15 pounds per square inch), a capacity which is slightly less than the strength of structural steel (~400 MPa). In addition to its incredible strength, hair also has elastic properties that enable it to stretch 20% of its original length when dry and up to 50% when wet. Given the tensile strength of each individual strand of hair, and the combined strength of thousands of hairs, this tissue is strong enough to support one's body weight – just ask Rapunzel! In fact, many Indian cultures used braided hair to make their ropes because of its strength and durability. Likewise, the Bible reminds us that, just like the hairs on our head, there is strength in numbers when we work as a team. For when we work together, we not only blend the knowledge and skills of many individuals, but our strength is magnified by a divine power that is greater than all of us.

This is true because if two or three people come together in my name, I am there with them (Matthew 18:20).

44

Amazing Maturity

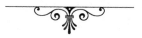

Hair color is the pigmentation of hair folli-cles due to two types of *melanin*: eumelanin and pheomelanin. Generally, when more melanin is present, the color of the hair is darker; if less melanin is present, the hair color is lighter. Pheomelanin colors hair red; all humans have some phoemelanin in their hair. Eumelanin, which has two subtypes of black or brown, determines the darkness of the hair color. A low concentration of brown eumelanin results in blond hair, whereas a higher concentration of brown eumel-anin will color the hair brown. High amounts of black eumelanin result in black hair, while low concentra-tions give us gray or white hair. Most people lose mel-anin as they age which triggers the graying process. Although popular culture may claim that blondes have more fun, brunettes are more intelligent, and redheads enjoy unbridled energy, the Book of Proverbs (16:31) suggests that it is those with gray hair ("a crown of glory") who lead a righteous life.

Interestingly, one of the latest fashion trends for hair seems to be to dye it gray. Perhaps these younger folks are seeking the virtue associated with this "crown of glory" or perhaps they are merely trying to imitate some silver-haired celebrities. Regardless of their motives, God will undoubtedly be able to distinguish those who are truly righteous from those who are not. And He has promised to care for His people, no matter how old or gray they become.

Family of Jacob, listen to me! All you people from Israel who are still alive, listen! I have carried you since you were born; I have taken care of you from your birth. Even when you are old, I will be the same. Even when your hair has turned gray, I will take care of you. I made you and will take care of you. I will carry you and save you (Isaiah 46:3-4).

45

Amazing Idiosyncrasy

*D*o you know which anatomical feature distinguishes primates from other mammals? Search the end of your fingers to find the answer. While most mammals have some type of claw at the end of their digits, primates have nails on their fingers and toes. Like hair, our nails are comprised primarily of a hardened protein called keratin. In addition to protein, nail strength is maintained by a diet that is enriched with calcium as well as vitamins B12 and C. A change in nail appearance is often a good indicator of some underlying pathology. For example, small pits in the fingernails may be an early sign of psoriasis; thick, yellowed nails are commonly associated with fungal infections; and dark stripes in the nail could suggest a form of melanoma (i.e., skin cancer). In addition, stress and lack of sleep can divert energy and nutrients away from the nails, slowing their growth rate. Normally, the average fingernail grows about 3.5 mm a month; that rate tends to be faster in the dominant hand, in men, and during the summer.

The Guinness world record for the longest set of fingernails currently belongs to Las Vegas singer, Christine Walton whose nails measure 10 feet and 2 inches (309.8 cm) on her left hand and 9 feet and 7 inches (292.1 cm) on her right hand for a combined length of 19 feet and 9 inches (601.9 cm). Ms. Walton seized the record from fellow American, Lee Redmond, whose fingernails reached a length of 28 feet and 4½ inches before she lost them in a 2009 auto accident. To get some perspective on these dimensions, imagine fingernails that are as long as a killer whale or the height of a two-story building. Although their long fingernails may have given these women a world record, this is not the sort of accomplishment that tends to enhance one's character. To accomplish that, we need to pursue goals that challenge us and make us stronger – as tough as nails! No matter what we choose as a career path, all of us are bound to encounter our share of hardship, criticism, or failure somewhere along the way. But just like a broken nail, we can grow from each of those experiences and be shaped into a better person. So embrace the adversity, and remember that triumph comes when we add a little *"umph"* to whatever we try.

For this reason I am happy when I have weaknesses, insults, hard times, sufferings, and all kinds of troubles for Christ. Because when I am weak, then I am truly strong (2 Corinthians 12:10).

46

Amazing Security

*O*ur bodies have many built-in defense mechanisms to protect us from the perils of our environment including our immune system and or sympathetic nervous system. But which organ is literally on the front line of our defense? If you said the skin, you would be absolutely correct! However, few of us typically think of our skin as a body organ even though it accounts for 15% of our total weight. For most people, that weight is heavier than the current Interceptor Body Armor System worn by U.S. military personnel. In addition to its weight, the skin covers a lot territory – as much as 22 square feet in some adults! Thus, this army of dermal cells provides a head-to-toe defense system that can ward off damaging ultraviolet rays and a host of invading bacteria. Much of the skin's defense mechanism is attributed to the acidic sweat and sebum on its surface that contain antibacterial and antifungal substances. Of course, these troops sustain a lot of casualties as we slough off about 30,000 to 40,000 skin cells every minute. This means that over his or her lifetime, the average human sheds about 40 pounds of skin! However, replacement troops are brought in almost as quickly as they are lost, so our skin's security remains intact. And although the skin is water resistant, its pores provide an outlet for many of the body's waste products which it excretes in the form of sweat. The cooling effect of this sweat, combined with the insulating effect of our triple-layered armor (epidermis, dermis, and subcutaneous tissues), helps regulate body temperature and maintain balance in our body fluids. But the skin's function does not end there. It also provides a home for a multitude of nerve endings which make the skin one of our primary sensory organs. These "special forces" enable us to perceive a variety of sensations ranging from a soothing caress or ticklish light touch to the pain of intense heat, cold, or pressure. Finally, the skin contributes to our identity through variations in its color, tone, wrinkles, scars, blemishes, and digital indentations that we recognize as hand and foot prints. So when it comes to physical protection, this marvelous, multi-faceted organ literally "has us covered." But when we need something more, it's nice to know we have a spiritual protector as well.

The Lord guards you. The Lord is the shade that protects you from the sun. The sun cannot hurt you during the day, and the moon cannot hurt you at night. The Lord will protect you from all dangers; he will guard your life. The Lord will guard you as you come and go, both now and forever (Psalm 121:5-8).

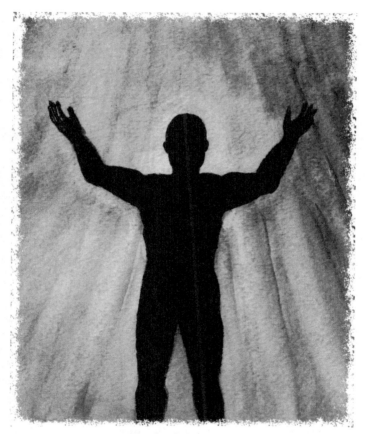

The body's armor

47

Amazing Discovery

Although the skin is remarkably resilient, when it is subjected to particularly harsh conditions such as burn trauma, it may be unable to adequately protect the tissues and organs that lie beneath it. Without the skin's protective armor, body temperature drops, fluids escape, and bacteria invades on a massive scale. Prior to the discovery and use of antibiotics, individuals with burn injuries over a large percentage of their skin surface usually died of hypovolemic shock or later succumbed to massive infection, a condition known as *sepsis*. But a tragic event in Boston, Massachusetts on November 28, 1942, changed medical history when physicians were faced with the unprecedented challenge of simultaneously treating hundreds of burn victims after a deadly fire broke out at the famous Cocoanut Grove nightclub. Like the perfect storm, this fire was fueled by a combination of factors including

the excessive use of highly flammable and toxic hol-
iday decorations, overcrowded conditions, a single
revolving door at the club's entrance, and obstructed
side exists (to discourage patrons from leaving without
paying their tab). As a result, 492 people lost their lives
when the fire broke out, and Boston's two major hospitals were overwhelmed with nearly 200 additional
burn victims that survived. But tragedy turned to triumph when the medical staff at Massachusetts General
Hospital used this disaster to pioneer new emergency
burn care procedures including fluid resuscitation,
blood transfusions, and less painful bandaging techniques. Although their innovative efforts saved many
lives initially, the threat of sepsis still loomed. And
then Merck and Company came to the rescue with
their donation of 32 liters of the recently developed
antibiotic, *penicillin!* This event marked the first use of
penicillin in the general population, and following its
success with the Cocoanut Grove fire victims, the U.S.
military ordered the immediate production and distri-
bution of penicillin to their armed forces. Undoubtedly
this wonder drug saved countless soldiers from similar
life-threatening injuries during the latter half of World
War II. But was the development of penicillin simply
good timing for these soldiers and civilians? As many
of them will attest, the real reason they were able to
overcome and survive such devastating injuries was
because God's protection stepped in when their body's
natural armor failed.

That is why you need to put on God's full armor. Then on the day of evil you will be able to stand strong. And when you have finished the whole fight, you will still be standing (Ephesians 6:13).

48

Amazing Viability

*O*n September 19, 1991, two German tourists stumbled onto the frozen remains of a 5,300-year old man who has since become known as "Ötzi, the Iceman." Ötzi's mummified body was found atop a 10,530 foot ridge in the Ötztal Alps, the mountains which form the border between Austria and Italy. Once archeologists extracted the body and determined its age, they launched what has been the most thorough forensic analysis performed on any corpse in recent history. Each investigative study has provided another piece of the puzzle revealing detailed information about this man's identity, lifestyle, and health status. The emerging picture is one of a 45-year old man who lived around 3300 BC, between the Copper and Bronze Ages. He was approximately 5'5" tall and probably weighed a little over 110 pounds. Using facial reconstruction technology, Ötzi's weathered appearance is depicted with deep-set brown eyes, sunken cheeks, straight brownish-gray hair and beard, and a variety of skin tattoos. Analysis of his hair and stomach contents indicated that Ötzi's diet consisted largely of meats and grains, and DNA analysis concluded that he was lactose intolerant. He apparently suffered from an intestinal parasite, several tooth cavities, atherosclerosis, and an early form of Lyme disease. The degenerative changes in his spine and lower extremity joints suggest that Ötzi did a lot of walking over hilly terrain and may have been a high-altitude shepherd. In 2012, Fox News reported that scientists had made another unusual discovery in Ötzi's body – it still contained intact red blood cells (RBCs). Given that these cells typically survive for no longer than 4 months, Ötzi's RBCs obviously set a new blood cell longevity record! But of all the secrets that have been revealed by Ötzi's autopsy, perhaps the most fascinating finding is that, more than 5,000 years later, he still has multiple living relatives. According to another 2012 news story published by the BBC, scientists affiliated with Innsbruck Medical University analyzed the DNA of more than 3,700 Austrian men from the region of Tyrol before identifying 19 who shared a somewhat rare genetic mutation with our famous Iceman. What are the odds of a single mutant gene remaining viable for more than 5 millennia? Obviously our bodies have many hidden secrets that even we are not aware of. Although science has developed sophisticated ways to predict our susceptibility to a variety of pathological conditions, perhaps there are times when it's better to be as uninformed as Ötzi was. After all, we shouldn't let the knowledge of our impending demise, get in the way of living the life God intended for us to enjoy.

> *So I decided it was more important to enjoy life. The best that people can do here on earth is to eat, drink, and enjoy life, because these joys will help them do the hard work God gives them here on earth (Ecclesiastes 8:15).*

49

Amazing Mortality

*H*ave you ever noticed the little plastic-coated tip at the end of a shoelace and thought about its function? Obviously, it makes it easier to thread the lace through the holes in our shoes, but it also prevents the ends of the shoelace from fraying and gradually becoming useless. Likewise, each strand of our DNA has a protective cap on both ends which is comprised of repetitive nucleotide sequences known as *telomeres* (from the Greek words for "end part").

Telomeres were first described in the mid-1970s by a trio of Harvard scientists who later won the 2009 Nobel Prize in Medicine for their discovery of how chromosomes are protected by these end structures. However, the role that telomeres play in the aging process was not well understood until more recently. We now know that when these telomeres become too short, they are unable to adequately protect the DNA from destructive chromosomal changes which affect the cell's ability to replicate. Without the ability to replicate, cells quickly age and die. Consequently, these senescent changes lead to deterioration of our organs and may result in a variety of age-related conditions such as cancer, diabetes, heart disease, osteoporosis, and dementia. An article published by Richard Cawthon in the February 2003 issue of *Lancet* was among the first to associate telomere shortening with higher mortality rates in humans. Thus, telomere shortening is like a ticking time clock that begins the countdown to our eventual demise as a human being. But what triggers this shortening and is there any way to prevent it? Recent studies have associated telomere shortening with unhealthy habits such as smoking, stress and anxiety, depression, and poor diets. Thus, people who pursue healthier lifestyles with regular physical exercise, reduced stress, and a diet rich in antioxidants, are more likely to retain greater telomere lengths.

However, there is yet another side to the telomere story. In addition to telomeres, scientists also discovered an enzyme called *telomerase* which can repair, and actually lengthen, the telomeres. Because the adult human has a very limited supply of telomerase (primarily in germ cells such as sperm and eggs), why don't we just find a way to synthesize it into a drug and distribute it as a universal cure for these age-related diseases? Obviously too much of a good thing has its drawbacks, and telomerase is no exception. The runaway growth of malignant cancer cells is one example.

These cells are rich in telomerase and largely unaffected by cellular aging. The debate on telomerase as the key to immortality will undoubtedly continue as scientists search for a biological "switch" that may control the activation of telomerase and maintain cell replication indefinitely. But is that really part of God's plan? The Bible clearly describes aging as a natural and inevitable process, one that eventually leads us to our "everlasting home." So perhaps we're better off letting those telomeres simply tick away.

Remember your Creator while you are young, before the days of trouble come and the years when you say, 'I find no pleasure in them.' When you get old, the light from the sun, moon, and stars will grow dark; the rain clouds will never seem to go away. At that time your arms will shake and your legs will become weak. Your teeth will fall out so you cannot chew, and your eyes will not see clearly. Your ears will be deaf to the noise in the streets, and you will barely hear the millstone grinding grain. You'll wake up when a bird starts singing, but you will barely hear singing. You will fear high places and will be afraid to go for a walk. Your hair will become white like the flowers on an almond tree. You will limp along like a grasshopper when you walk. Your appetite will be gone. Then you will go to your everlasting home, and people will go to your funeral (Ecclesiastes 12:1-5).

50

Amazing Longevity

*A*lthough we now know that telomere length of DNA affects the rate of aging and limits our lifespan, there is still considerable debate among the scientific community regarding human longevity. Scientists now conclude that the maximum lifespan for the average human in no more than 120 years, a time at which cell division seems to stop. Basically, it is the "end of the line" for those telomeres which can shorten no more. Interestingly, 120 is the same number of years that God said he would allow man to live as recorded in Genesis: *"The Lord said, 'My Spirit will not remain in human beings forever, because they are flesh. They will live only 120 years.'"* (Genesis 6:3)

So how do we account for Old Testament records of people like Adam, Noah, Methuselah, and others whose lifespans exceeded 900 years? In fact, the first three books of the Bible document 28 individuals who lived well beyond 120 years. Yet, by the time David wrote the Book of Psalms, the predicted lifespan had already diminished to a number that is similar to current census statistics of 78.7 years:

Our lifetime is seventy years or, if we are strong, eighty years. But the years are full of hard work and pain. They pass quickly, and then we are gone (Psalm 90:10).

At what point did things change and why? Some theologians and scientists speculate that when God decided to destroy the earth with the great flood, he also instilled some type of DNA mutation that gradually accelerated the aging process in all future generations. The point at which our bodies begin to deteriorate with age is also known as *senescence*. Indirectly, senescence is the leading cause of death in humans. According to a 2007 article published by Aubrey de Grey of the Methuselah Foundation, aging kills about 100,000 people a day worldwide (approximately 2/3 of the total). In industrialized nations that proportion is even higher, climbing to 90%! However, we rarely see "old age" listed as the cause of death on certificates issued in the U.S. Instead we will see conditions such as heart disease, stroke, renal failure, or other disorders that relate to senescence of various body organs.

Although senescence is not unique to the human organism, there are a few plant and animal species that seem to defy the odds when it comes to the aging process. In addition to trees like the bristlecone pine and giant sequoia which live for thousands of years, scientists have documented some species of crabs, clams, turtles, lizards, whales, koi (fish), sea urchins, and jellyfish that may live for hundreds of years. The relatively isolated and stress-free environment that these animals inhabit seems to support the philosophy of "live slow, live long." Whether they effectively avoid the stressors that accelerate senescence or are simply more resilient to its effects, we could probably all learn a lesson from their lifestyle. So don't be afraid to slow down once in a while, leave the stress behind, and move at the pace of an old tortoise. Not only are we likely to live longer, but we will indeed become wiser.

Teach us how short our lives really are so that we may be wise (Psalm 90:12).

51

Amazing Capability

*D*o you remember a game show that aired a few years ago on TV called *"Who wants to be a millionaire?"* In order to win the grand prize, contestants had to select the correct answer to 15 increasingly difficult, multiple-choice questions. When the contestant got stuck on a question, he or she had the option of using one of three available "lifelines" including "ask the audience," "50/50" (narrowed the possibilities by half), or "phone a friend." Sometimes these lifelines saved a contestant, but just as often, they failed. Fortunately the first lifeline we are given is much more reliable. That lifeline is our *umbilical cord*. This 20-inch connection between the mother's placenta and the baby's stomach provides all the nourishment and oxygen that the fetus needs to fully develop until it is ready to live on its own. Interestingly, the umbilical cord contains one vein and two arteries that seem to function in reverse of what we typically see these blood vessels doing after birth. The umbilical vein sends fresh, oxygenated blood to the fetus while the two arteries remove blood that is filled with carbon dioxide and waste products. Shortly after birth, the umbilical cord is clamped and cut, forcing the newborn to "fend for itself" as an independent organism. The umbilical cord is typically discarded, although many of these structures are now being saved in tissue banks where their stem cells may later be harvested and used to help treat a variety of degenerative diseases. But basically, once the child has been delivered, the work of the umbilical cord is done. It has served its one important purpose. Likewise, each of us is given a job to do, and we must do it to the best of our ability. Some of us will save lives on a daily basis, while others will deal with tragic deaths. Many will provide comfort and hope to those who are suffering from devastating injuries or disease. But all of us will encounter some rewards along our career path, often at the most unexpected times.

As a physical therapist I have experienced many of these precious moments. I can recall one patient who was recovering from a neurological condition known as Guillain-Barré Syndrome. This disease, thought to be triggered by a viral infection, causes a progressive weakness or paralysis down the extremities. After a period of time, the nerves gradually regenerate, and the person usually regains most of the sensory and motor function that he or she had lost. Although this particular patient was in the recovery phase of her disease, her progress was very slow, and she was still experiencing significant weakness and balance problems. The sensation in her lower legs and feet was still impaired, and she had no response to reflex testing. Then one day, it happened. I tapped her patellar tendon, and we saw a slight knee jerk. Just a tiny movement, but it symbolized a huge milestone in her recovery process. What joy was in the room! She and her husband embraced, kissed, and celebrated this long-awaited sign as if they had just won the lottery. And maybe they did. I did nothing but elicit the response with my reflex hammer; God had already performed His miracle. But seeing such little things make such a big difference in someone's life – that is the ultimate reward of caring for the human body!

If we pay close attention, all of us will experience a lifetime of rewards for our work. And as Christian believers, we have been given a second lifeline through the gift of the Holy Spirit which cannot be severed. It will forever connect us to the power that helps us grow and learn as we care for His most precious creation – the human body.

In all the work you are doing, work the best you can. Work as if you were doing it for the Lord, not for people. Remember that you will receive your reward from the Lord, which he promised to his people. You are serving the Lord Christ (Colossians 3:23-24).

52

Amazing Unity

$\mathcal{R}$emember earlier when we talked about the frog's inability to hop backwards due to the limitations of its vestibular system? And yet that same frog can catch a flying insect in mid-air with its tongue which requires a reaction time that is far faster than the human eye can see. So we might wonder, *"Who cares? Humans don't need to catch flying insects with their tongues!"* Likewise, a frog doesn't need to hop backwards. So obviously we are all endowed by our Creator with different anatomical designs and physio-logical abilities based upon our unique purpose in life and what we need to grow and thrive. Although there are structural and functional variations in every plant and animal species, the variability among humans is probably the most pronounced even though we all share similar anatomical components. Our differences lie in the gifts we are given and how we use those gifts to fulfill our common purpose – to care for one another. So whether one's life calling is in one of the health care professions, teaching, law enforcement, counseling, ministry, computer technology, business, entertainment, cleaning and maintenance, or some other type of work, each of us have been given a special gift that can be used to fulfill that common purpose. As each of us develops our gifts, I hope we will keep in mind the following scriptural passage where the Apostle Paul uses the human body to remind us that we all have an equally important role to play in pursuit of this shared purpose. And with God's spirit to guide us, we cannot fail.

A person's body is one thing, but it has many parts. Though there are many parts to a body, all those parts make only one body. Christ is like that also. Some of us are Jews, and some are Greeks. Some of us are slaves, and some are free. But we were all baptized into one body through one Spirit. And we were all made to share in the one Spirit. The human body has many parts. The foot might say, 'Because I am not a hand, I am not part of the body.' But saying this would not stop the foot from being a part of the body. The ear might say, "Because I am not an eye, I am not part of the body." But saying this would not stop the ear from being a part of the body. If the whole body were an eye, it would not be able to hear. If the whole body were an ear, it would not be able to smell.

If each part of the body were the same part, there would be no body. But truly God put all the parts, each one of them, in the body as he wanted them. So then there are many parts, but only one body (1 Corinthians 12:12-20).

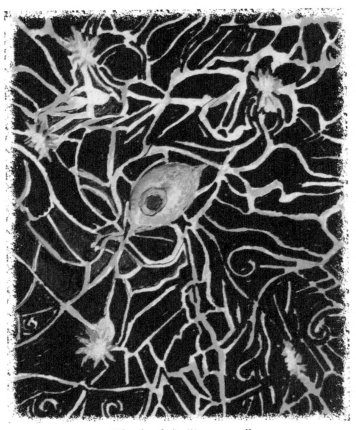

The body's "intranet"

AFTERWORD
FOR TEACHERS

*T*he idea for this book originated from my experience as a professor of physical therapy at Hardin-Simmons University, a faith-based institution located in Abilene, Texas. I have been blessed further with encouragement from many professional colleagues across the country as I completed this project. Although we all strive for excellence in our teaching, it is often difficult to define what that means and how to best accomplish it. But the Apostle Paul told us in his letter to the Corinthians, *"I will show you the most excellent way."* In the chapter that follows (I Corinthians 13) Paul writes some of the most eloquent and frequently-cited verses in the Bible where he defines excellence in terms of love. I have taken the liberty to adapt this famous scriptural passage for my fellow teachers as a reminder of the important role they play in shaping the lives of future health care providers. Regardless of the subject we teach, our work is bound to be excellent if it is grounded in love.

If I could explain everything perfectly to my students, but did not love each one of them, I might as well be talking to empty chairs. And if I knew all the answers to their questions and had evidence to support everything I teach but did not demonstrate love, my efforts would be worthless. If I could have the latest educational technology to equip my classroom, but did not use it with love, it would be a complete waste. Love is patient when it must repeat a concept over and over to a student who has difficulty grasping it. Love keeps trying when a student struggles to understand the complexities of human physiology or dilemmas of health care ethics. Love is kind when a student needs extra guidance to learn a new manual skill or encouragement to perform better on the next exam. Love is not jealous when students praise another teacher's course, nor boastful when they express appreciation for what they've learned in mine. Love does not delight in students' failures, but rejoices in their successes. Love bears all negativities, believes in all possibilities, hopes for all opportunities, and endures all difficulties. Love never ends. As for knowledge, it will pass away; our textbooks and research will become obsolete.

But the wisdom and experience I have gained are everlasting. So these three things I have learned from teaching: persistence, patience, and love. But the greatest of these is love.

Dr. Martha R. Hinman

ABOUT THE ARTIST
AND ILLUSTRATIONS

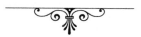

*M*aria del Carmen Cabrera is an artist who currently resides in Mission, Texas. After earning her baccalaureate degree in Art and Spanish from the Texas A&M University in Kingsville, Ms. Cabrera attended graduate school at the Academy of San Carlos in Mexico City as well as Texas A&M in Kingsville. During her 30-year career as an art teacher, Ms. Cabrera has inspired hundreds of junior high and high school students, many of whom later pursued their own artistic careers. Although she uses a variety of media in her artwork, Ms. Cabrera's favorite medium is watercolor which she selected to illustrate *Amazing Grays*. Additional media such as colored pencils were used to enhance the detail and clarity of these anatomical drawings.

In their order of appearance, the illustrations in this book include the following: a sperm fertilizing an egg, cross-section of a knee joint, the four chambers of the heart, the heart and lungs, close-up of an eye, a nerve cell (neuron), the brain, a man reaching upward (stretching his skin), and a network of neurons synapsing with one another.

BIBLIOGRAPHY

Books, Magazines, Special Reports

Barnes, Jeffrey G. "History." In *Fingerprint Sourcebook*, by International Association for Identification, pp. 1-18. (Washington, DC: U.S. Department of Justice, 2011). Accessed September 9, 2015, https://www.ncjrs.gov/pdf-files1/nij/ 235392.pdf.

Berens EM. *A Handbook of Mythology: Myths and Legends of Ancient Greece and Rome (1886)* (New York, NY: Kessinger Publishing, 2008), 20

Carter, Rita. *The Human Brain Book.* (New York, NY: Dorling Kindersley Ltd., 2009).

Challoner, Jack. *Amazing Body Facts and Trivia.* (New York, NY: Chartwell Books, Inc., 2011).

Christian, Frank. *A Scientist's View of the Bible and More*. (Bloomington, IN: WestBow Press, 2011).

Cutter, Mary Ann G, et al. *Mapping and Sequencing the Human Genome: Science, Ethics, and Public Policy*. (Colorado Springs, CO: Biological Sciences Curriculum Study, 1992.) Accessed September 9, 2015, http://files.eric.ed.gov/fulltext/ED462289.pdf

Daniels, Patricia. *The Body: A Complete User's Guide*. (Washington DC: National Geographic, 2014).

Gregorc, Anthony F. *An Adult's Guide to Style*. (Columbia, CT: Gregorc Associates, 1982).

Hayes, Bill. *The Anatomist: A True Story of Gray's Anatomy*. New York, NY: Bellevue Literary Press, 2009).

Keyes, Edward. *Cocoanut Grove*. (New York, NY: Atheneum, 1984).

Kosslun, Steven M. and G. Wayne Miller. *Top Brain, Bottom Brain: Harnessing the Power of the Four Cognitive Modes*, 2nd edition. (New York, NY: Simon and Schuster, 2015).

McCutcheon, Marc. *The Compass in Your Nose and Other Astonishing Facts About Humans*. (Los Angeles: Jeremy P. Tarcher Inc., 1989).

Newsweek Special Issue. *Your Body*. (New York, NY: Topix Meida Lab, Sept/Oct 2014).

Pronovost, Peter and Eric Vohr. *Safe Patients, Smart Hospitals*. (New York, NY: Hudson Street Press, 2010), 46.

Seuling, Barbara. *Your Skin Weighs More Than Your Brain and Other Freaky Facts About Your Skin, Skeleton, and Other Body Parts*. (Minneapolis, MN: Picture Window Books, 2008).

Journal Articles

Beck, Konrad, Irene Hunter, Jurgen Engel. "Structure and function of laminin: anatomy of a multidomain glycoprotein." *The FASEB Journal* 4 no. 2 (1990): 148-160.

Brown, Christopher A., Aijing Z. Starr, James A. Nunley. "Analysis of past secular trends of hip fractures and predicted number in the future 2010–2050." *Journal of Orthopaedic Trauma* 26 no. 2 (2012): 117–122.

Cawthon, Richard M, et al. "Association between telomere length in blood and mortality in people aged 60 years or older." *Lancet* 361 (2003): 393-395.

Chahal, Harvinder S, et al. "AIP mutation in pituitary adenomas in the 18th century and today." *New England Journal of Medicine* 364 no. 1 (2011): 43-50.

Chen, Thomas S. N. and Peter S. Y. Chen. "The myth of Prometheus and the liver." *Journal of the Royal Society of Medicine* 87 no. 12 (1994): 754–755.

De Grey, Aubrey D. N. J. "Life span extension research and public debate: Societal considerations." *Studies in Ethics, Law, and Technology* 1 (2015): Article 5. Accessed September 15, 2015. http://www.sens.org/files/pdf/ENHANCE-PP.pdf

Dias, Brian G., and Kerry J. Ressler. "Parental olfactory experience influences behavior and neural structure in subsequent generations." *Nature Neuroscience* 17, no. 1 (2014): 89-96.

Dijkstra, Katinka; Michael P. Kaschak, Rolf A.Zwaan. "Body posture facilitates retrieval of autobiographical memories." *Cognition* 102 no. 1 (2007): 139-149.

Dote K, et al. "Myocardial stunning due to simultaneous multivessel coronary spasms: A review of 5 cases." *Journal of Cardiology* 21 no. 2 (1991): 203-214.

Dy, Christopher J., et al. "An economic evaluation of a systems-based strategy to expedite surgical treatment of hip fractures" [published correction appears in *Journal of Bone & Joint Surgery, American Volume* 93 no. 14 (2011):1334]. *Journal of Bone & Joint Surgery, American Volume* 93 no. 14 (2011):1326–1334.

Edwards, William D, Wesley J. Gabel, Floyd E. Hosmer. "On the physical death of Jesus Christ." *JAMA* 255 no. 11 (1986): 1455-1463.

Evinger, Craig. "A brain stem reflex in the blink of an eye." *News in Physiological Sciences* 10 no. 4 (1995): 147-153.

Kuilman, Thomas, Chrysiis Michaloglou, Wolter J. Mooi, Daniel S. Peeper. "The essence of senescence." *Genes and Development* 24 no. 22 (2010): 2463-2479.

Komisaruk, Barry R., et al. "Women's clitoris, vagina, and cervix mapped on the sensory cortex: fMRI evidence." *The Journal of Sexual Medicine* 8 no. 10 (2011): 2822-2830.

LeBlanc, Kim E.; Herbert L. Muncie Jr, Leanne L. LeBlanc. "Hip fracture: Diagnosis, treatment, and secondary prevention." *American Family Physician* 89 no. 12 (2014): 945-951.

Lopez, Alan D. et al. "Global and regional burden of disease and risk factors, 2001: systematic analysis of population health data." *Lancet* 367 (2006): 1747-1757.

Maslen, Matthew W. and Peirs D. Mitchell. "Medical theories on the cause of death in crucifixion." *Journal of the Royal Society of Medicine* 99 no. 4 (2006): 185-188.

Mitchell, H. H., T. S. Hamilton, F. R. Steggerda, and H. W. Bean. "The chemical composition of the adult human body and its bearing on the biochemistry of growth." *Journal of Biological Chemistry* 158 (1945): 625-637.

Nielsen, Jared A., et al. "An evaluation of the left-brain vs. right-brain hypothesis with resting state functional connectivity magnetic resonance imaging." *PLoS ONE* 8 (2013): e71275, accessed September 15, 2015, doi:10.1371/journal.pone.0071275.

Ochs, Matthias, et al. "The number of alveoli in the human lung." *American Journal of Respiratory and Critical Care Medicine* 169 no. 1 (2004): 120-124.

Pearsall, Paul, Gary E. R. Schwartz, Linda G. S. Russek. "Changes in heart transplant recipients that parallel the personalities of their donors."

Journal of Near-Death Studies 20 no. 3 (2002): 191-2006.

Rizvi, Saliha, Syed T. Raza and Farzana Mahdi "Telomere length variations in aging and age-related diseases." *Current Aging Science* 7 no. 3 (2014): 161-167

Singh, Kuljit, et al. "Meta-analysis of clinical correlates of acute mortality in Takotsubo cardiomyopathy." *The American Journal of Cardiology* 113 no. 8 (2014): 1420-1428.

Snowdon, David A. "Aging and Alzheimer's disease: Lessons from the Nun Study." *The Gerontologist* 37 no. 2 (1997): 150-156.

Snowdon, David A. "Healthy aging and dementia: Findings from the Nun Study." *Annals of Internal Medicine* 139 no. 5 (2003): 450-454.

Wang, ZiMian, et al. "Hydration of fat-free body mass: review and critique of a classic body-composition constant." *The American Journal of Clinical Nutrition* 69 no. 5 (1999): 833-841.

Websites

Andras, Simon. "20 amazing facts about dreams that you might not know about." Accessed September 9, 2015. http://www.lifehack.org/articles/

productivity/20-amazing-facts-about-dreams-that-you-might-not-know-about.html.

Baidya, Sankalan. "35 facts about human kidneys." Last update April 18, 2015. Accessed September 9, 2015. http://factslegend. org/35-facts-human-kidneys/.

BBC News. "Link to Oetzi the Iceman found in living Austrians." Last updated October 10, 2013. Accessed September 9, 2015. http://www.bbc. com/ news/world-europe-24477038.

Centers for Medicare and Medicaid Services. "National health expenditures 2013 highlights." Accessed September 9, 2015, https:// www.cms.gov/ Research-Statistics-Data-and-Systems/Statistics-Trends-and-Reports/National HealthExpendData/ downloads/highlights.pdf.

"Human Longevity Facts." Accessed September 8, 2015, http://myth-one.com/chapter_19.htm.

Christiensen, Vickie. "What is the stapedius?" Last updated July 24, 2015. Accessed September 9, 2015, http://www.wisegeek.com/what-is-the-stapedius.htm.

Cleveland Clinic. "What your tongue can tell you about your health." Last updated April 27, 2015. Accessed September 9, 2015, http://health.

cleveland clinic.org/2015/04/what-your-tongue-can-tell-you-about-your-health/.

"Cocoanut Grove fire." In *Wikipedia*. Last modified on September 5, 2015. https://en.wikipedia.org/wiki/Cocoanut_Grove_fire.

"Compilation of 15 speeds records." Last updated June 14, 2009. Accessed September 9, 2015, http://www.supertightstuff.com/06/14/motoring/compilation-of-15-speed-records/.

Discovery Eye Foundation. "20 facts about the amazing eye." Last updated June 10, 2014. Accessed September 9, 2015, http://discoveryeye.org/blog/20-facts-about-the-amazing-eye/.

Erens, Greg A, Thomas S. Thornhill, and Jeffrey N. Katz. "Total hip arthroplasty." Last updated February 10, 2015. Accessed September 9, 2015, http://www.uptodate.com/contents/total-hip-arthroplasty.

Foster, Katherine W. "Hip fractures in adults." Last updated March 31, 2015. Accessed September 9, 2015, http://www.uptodate.com/contents/hip-fractures-in-adults#H2.

Georgia State University. "Rods and cones." Accessed September 8, 2015, http://hyperphysics.phy-astr.gsu.edu/hbase/vision/rodcone.html.

Gewin, V. "Not all species deteriorate with age." Last updated December
8, 2013. Accessed September 9,
2015, http://www.nature.com/ news/
not-all-species-deteriorate-with-age-1.14322.

Gillin, J. Christian. "How long can humans stay
awake?" Last updated March 25, 2002. Accessed
September 9, 2015, http://www.scientificamer-
ican. com/article/how-long-can-humans-stay/.

Global Security. "Interceptor body armor." Accessed
September 9, 2015, http://www.globalsecurity.
org/military/systems/ground/interceptor.htm

Guinness World Records. "Largest natural breasts."
Last updated January 1, 1999. Accessed
September 8, 2015, http://www.guinnessworldre-
cords.com/ world-records/largest-natural-breasts.

Guinness World Records. "Record holder pro-
file: Christine Walton – owner of the world's
longest fingernails." Last updated September
14, 2011. Accessed September 8, 2015,
http://www.guinness worldrecords.com/
news/2011/9/record-holder-profile-chris-
tine-walton-%E2%80%93-owner-of-the-
world%E2%80%99s-longest-fingernails/.

Hiskey, Daven. "Charles Osborne had the hiccups for 68 years, from 1922 to 1990." Last

updated July 19, 2011. Accessed September 8, 2015, http://www. todayifoundout.com/index. php/2011/07/charles-osborne-had-the-hiccups-for-68-years-from-1922-to-1990/.

"Human hair color." In *Wikipedia*. Last modified September 7, 2015. https://en.wikipedia.org/wiki/ Human_hair_color.

Jenkins, Beverly. "Fart Facts: 10 facts about farting." Last updated December 24, 2014). Accessed September 9, 2015, http://www.oddee.com/ item_98612.aspx.

Kaltenborn, Freddy. "Ancient roots of joint traction." Last updated November 2, 2014. Accessed September 8, 2015, http://www.freddykaltenborn. com/category/history/.

National Kidney Foundation. "Kidney disease." Accessed September 9, 2015, https://www. kidney.org/kidneydisease/.

Nestle. "Water in your body." Accessed September 9, 2015, http://www.nestle-waters.com/ healthy-hydration/water-body.

Neurogistics, Inc. "What are neurotransmitters?" Accessed September 9, 2015, https:// www. neurogistics.com/TheScience/ WhatareNeurotransmi09CE.asp.

"Nine things you never knew about sperm." Last updated November 20, 2013. Accessed September 9, 2015, http://www.huffingtonpost. com/2013/ 11/20/nine-things-you-never-knew-about-sperm-photos_n_4268031.html.

Osborn, David. "Achilles and his vulnerable heel." Accessed September 9, 2015, http://www.greek medicine.net/mythology/achilles.html.

"tzi." In *Wikipedia*. Last modified August 27, 2015. https://en.wikipedia.org/wiki/%C3%96tzi/.

Pappas, S. "'Iceman' mummy holds world's oldest blood cells." Last updated May 2, 2013. Accessed September 9, 2015, http:// www.foxnews.com/ scitech/2012/05/02/ iceman-mummy-holds-world-oldest-blood-cells/.

Premier Exhibitions, Inc. "Edentulous: a brief history of dentures." Accessed September 9, 2015, http://www.premierexhibitions. com/exhibitions/4/4/bodies-exhibition/blog/ edentulous-brief-history-dentures.

Reader's Digest. "13 of your most embarrassing health questions answered." Accessed September 9, 2015, http://www.rd.com/health/wellness/13-of-your-most-embarrassing-health-questions-answered/.

Roberts, Jeff. "There's an organ in your brain which seats your soul: Meet your pineal gland." Last updated December 15, 2013. Accessed September 9, 2015, http://www. collective-evolution.com/2013/ 12/15/ theres-an-organ-in-your-brain-which-seats-your-soul-meet-your-pineal-gland/.

Salemi, V. "New survey shows smiling is the best way to make a first impression." Last updated February 26, 2013. Accessed September 9, 2015, http://www.adweek.com/fishbowlny/new-survey-shows-smiling-is-the-best-way-to-make-a-first-impression/322531?red=mj.

Schocker, Laura. "15 Things you never knew about your nails." Last updated September 24, 2013. Accessed September 9, 2015, http://www.huff-ington post.com/2013/09/24/nail-facts-finger-nails_n_ 3957467.html.

Sinclair Intimacy Institute. "Breasts." Last updated April 25, 2005. Accessed September 9, 2015, http://health.howstuffworks.com/sexual-health/ female-reproductive-system/breasts-dictio-nary1.htm.

Thurtle, Estelle. "10 Unnerving premonitions that foretold disaster." Last updated April 9, 2014. Accessed September 9, 2015, http://listverse.

com/ 2014/04/28/10-unnerving-premoni-
tions-that-foretold-disaster/.

Turner, Rebecca. "The man who never slept."
Accessed September 9, 2015, http://www.world-
of-lucid-dreaming.com/the-man-who-never-
slept.html.

U.S. Environmental Protection Agency. "Overview
of greenhouse gases: methane emissions."
Accessed September 8, 2015, http://www.
epa.gov/climate change/ghgemissions/gases/
ch4.html.

Vey, Gary. "The pineal gland—the 'seat of the soul'?"
Accessed September 8, 2015, http://www.view-
zone.com/pineal.html.

WebMD. "Eye health center." Accessed September
8, 2015, http://www.webmd.com/eye-health/
picture-of-the-eyes.

Weizmann Institute. "Sperm use heat sensors to find the egg." Last updated
February 3, 2003. Accessed September
9, 2015, http://www.sciencedaily.com/
releases/2003/02/030203071703.htm.

CPSIA information can be obtained at www.ICGtesting.com
Printed in the USA
BVOW11s1331141215

430241BV00015B/622/P

9 781498 456685